The Metabolic Syndrome: The Road Map from Inflammation to Cardiovascular Disease

The Metabolic Syndrome: The Road Map from Inflammation to Cardiovascular Disease

Proceedings of the 9th European Symposium on Metabolism
held in Padua, Italy, between 12 and 14 October 2006

Editors:

Gaetano Crepaldi
C.N.R. – Center of Aging
University of Padua
Padua, Italy

Antonio Tiengo
Department of Clinical and Experimental Medicine
Metabolic Diseases
University of Padua
Padua, Italy

Angelo Avogaro
Department of Clinical and Experimental Medicine
Metabolic Diseases
University of Padua
Padua, Italy

ELSEVIER
2007

ELSEVIER B.V.
Radarweg 29
P.O. Box 211, 1000 AE Amsterdam
The Netherlands

ELSEVIER Inc.
525 B Street, Suite 1900
San Diego, CA 92101-4495
USA

ELSEVIER Ltd
The Boulevard, Langford Lane
Kidlington, Oxford OX5 1GB
UK

ELSEVIER Ltd
84 Theobalds Road
London WC1X 8RR
UK

First edition 2007

Library of Congress Cataloging in Publication Data
A catalog record from the Library of Congress has been applied for.

British Library Cataloguing in Publication Data
A catalogue record from the British Library has been applied for.

International Congress Series No. 1303
ISBN-13: 978-0-444-52889-6
ISBN-10: 0-444-52889-X
ISSN: 0531-5131

∞ The paper used in this publication meets the requirements of ANSI/NISO Z39.48-1992 (Permanence of Paper).

Transferred to Digital Printing 2009.

Acknowledgements

The editors gratefully acknowledge the efforts of the numerous speakers at the 9th European Symposium on Metabolism held in Padua (Italy) in October 2006 who prepared the edited version of their presentations now appearing in this volume.

Introduction

Based on the Proceedings of the 9th European Symposium on Metabolism held in Padua (Italy) in October 2006, this reference book reflects the latest research findings on the metabolic syndrome, an association of metabolic and hemodynamic alterations causing a predisposition for atherosclerosis and explaining the rising increase in death and morbidity due to cardiovascular diseases. Collecting the contribution of the most renown experts in the field of genetics, epidemiology, and physiopathology, the symposium focused on the role of oxidative stress and of endothelial dysfunction on the development of atherosclerosis. Abdominal obesity, pro-inflammatory adipokines and atherogenesis, cadiovascular global risk, coronary and cerebrovascular disease, the management, prevention and treatment of the metabolic syndrome and its cardiovascular complications were the major topics that were dealt with and examined during the course of the symposium.

This volume will prove without doubt to be a useful aid to practitioners and specialists striving to prevent and to treat the metabolic syndrome and its complications in their diabetic and cardiac patients.

ELSEVIER

International Congress Series 1303 (2007) vii

www.ics-elsevier.com

Preface

This collection of papers represents an edited version of the Proceedings of the 9th European Symposium on Metabolism which was held at the University of Padua (Italy) from October 12–14, 2006.

As did the Symposium itself, this work unites under a single cover topics dealing with four important metabolic alterations: diabetes, obesity, hyperlipidemia and hypertension. Of vital interest to the scientific community because of their cost in human life and medical expenditure, the latest edition of this Symposium received much attention from investigators in these fields.

The 2006 edition focused on the most recent epidemiologic findings on the role of oxidative stress and of endothelial dysfunction on the development of atherosclerosis. Other topics of particular interest were: abdominal obesity, pro-inflammatory adipokines and atherogenesis; the metabolic syndrome and cardiovascular global risk; coronary and cerebrovascular disease in diabetes and in the metabolic syndrome. Finally, the management, prevention and treatment of the metabolic syndrome and its cardiovascular complications were examined in the light of several recent clinical trials in these fields.

Moreover, the G. B. Morgagni Prizes, supported by an unrestricted educational grant by Servier and presented under the auspices of the Faculty of Medicine of the University of Padua, were once again associated to the symposium's program. During the Awards Ceremony, held within the context of the Symposium, the 2006 G. B. Morgagni Medal was awarded to Dr. Gerd Assmann from München (Germany) for his outstanding research in the field of lipoprotein metabolism and atherosclerosis prevention. His Morgagni Medal Lecture, "The role of genetic disposition and biomarkers in atherosclerosis", will be published in an upcoming issue of the *European Journal of Clinical Investigation*. But I would like to point out that Dr. Assmann had already been invited to speak at our meeting even before the qualifications of the candidates were evaluated and that is why you will find a paper by him on phytosterols and atherosclerosis that was likewise presented during the symposium.

This volume will certainly be of interest to all those practitioners and specialists who are looking for a broad, though specific overview on several aspects of insulin resistance as a possible pathogenetic mechanism and a guide to preventing and treating the metabolic syndrome and its cardiovascular complications in their patients.

Gaetano Crepaldi
Chairman of the 9th European Symposium on Metabolism
Padua, Italy, December 2006

doi:10.1016/j.ics.2007.01.065

Contents

Is the Metabolic Syndrome still alive?

International Congress Series 1303 (2007) 3–9

www.ics-elsevier.com

The metabolic syndrome: Is it still alive?

Enzo Bonora *

Endocrinology and Metabolism, University of Verona, Italy

Abstract. The metabolic syndrome is very common in the general population and is defined by the clustering of several cardiovascular risk factors, such as type 2 diabetes, hypertension, high triglyceride and low high density lipoprotein cholesterol. Central obesity and insulin resistance are underlying disorders of the syndrome as well as further risk factors for cardiovascular disease. Moreover, a panel of novel, non-traditional risk factors are ancillary features of the metabolic syndrome. They include biomarkers of chronic mild inflammation (e.g., C-reactive protein), oxidant stress (e.g., oxidized low density lipoprotein), thrombophilia (e.g., Plasminogen Activator Inhibitor-1), abnormal adipocyte activity (e.g., adiponectin), and endothelial dysfunction (e.g., E-selectin). Therefore, subjects with the metabolic syndrome are potentially at high risk of developing atherosclerosis and clinical cardiovascular events. In recent years several longitudinal studies have confirmed that subjects with the metabolic syndrome present with atherosclerosis and suffer from myocardial infarction and stroke at rates higher than subjects without the syndrome. The risk of cardiovascular disease is particularly high in women with the syndrome and in subjects with pre-existing diabetes and cardiovascular disease. However, an increased risk is already present in subjects with a cluster of multiple mild abnormalities. The risk related to the metabolic syndrome is definitely higher when subjects affected are compared to subjects free of any metabolic abnormality. Although many aspects related to the metabolic syndrome need to be better elucidated, and several concerns recently raised about the syndrome need to be adequately addressed by further investigations, the clinical value of identifying subjects with this common metabolic condition seems fully valid. © 2007 Published by Elsevier B.V.

Keywords: Metabolic syndrome; Central obesity; Insulin resistance; Dyslipidemia; Hypertension; Type 2 diabetes mellitus; Cardiovascular disease

* Endocrinologia e Metabolismo, Università di Verona, Ospedale Maggiore, Piazzale Stefani, 1, 37126 Verona, Italy. Tel.: +39 045 812 3113; fax: +39 045 917374.

E-mail addresses: enzobonora@virgilio.it, enzo.bonora@univr.it.

doi:10.1016/j.ics.2007.03.020

1. Historical background and size of the clinical problem

It is well known that metabolic disorders such as type 2 diabetes (T2DM), dyslipidemia, hyperuricemia, obesity and hypertension often cluster in the same individual. The first descriptions in the literature of what nowadays is called metabolic syndrome came from Kylin in Sweden [1], Vague in France [2], and Avogaro and co-workers in Italy [3]. A fundamental impulse in the development of the pathophysiological concepts surrounding the metabolic syndrome and in the research in this field came from Reaven, who was the first to provide a nosologic dignity and a name to the syndrome [4]. In subsequent years other investigators focused on the cluster, appealing it with several different names and suggesting different diagnostic approaches [5–9]. At the end of the past decade the World Health Organization (WHO) appointed a group of experts who were committed to identify the most appropriate diagnostic criteria of the syndrome [10]. The criteria established by this working group, however, required an intriguing and not feasible assessment of insulin resistance by the glucose clamp. Mainly for such reason other groups of experts, appointed by the National Cholesterol Education Program–Adult Panel Treatment III (NCEP–ATPIII), the American Heart Association and the National Heart, Lung and Blood Institute (AHA-NHBLI), and the International Diabetes Federation (IDF), suggested a more clinically oriented approach, based upon the assessment of parameters easily available for any physician and easier to standardize [11–13]. Unfortunately, these criteria were somewhat inconsistent and, therefore, a certain degree of confusion still exists when one aims at identifying subjects with the metabolic syndrome.

Whatever are the diagnostic criteria used, population-based study clearly documented that the metabolic syndrome is very common [14–17], although the overlap between affected subjects identified with the different sets of diagnostic criteria is only partial. Fig. 1 illustrates the prevalence of the metabolic syndrome in the general population aged 40–79 years living in Bruneck, north-eastern Italy. The prevalence ranged from 17.5% with NCEP-ATPIII criteria to 33.5% with IDF criteria.

2. The Metabolic Syndrome Paradox

The interest surrounding the metabolic syndrome is sizable, with more than 5000 papers published in the scientific literature including this term in the title and/or the abstract. As a consequence, the knowledge on the syndrome has dramatically grown in the last two decades. When Reaven in 1988 described Syndrome X [4], the etiopathogenesis was poorly

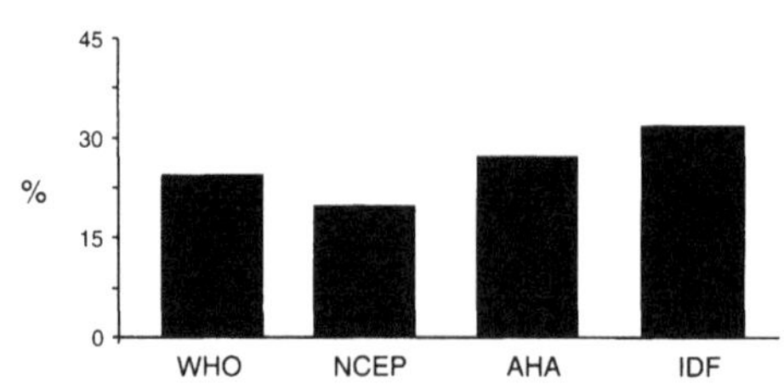

Fig. 1. Prevalence of the metabolic syndrome in the Bruneck Study according to current diagnostic criteria. Bruneck Study, $n=919$, age 40–79 years (Bonora et al, unpublished data).

defined, the clinical features were not fully understood, and the outcome was only postulated. At that time the criteria required for the existence of a disease/syndrome were not satisfied. At present these criteria are met because a bulk of experimental data indicated that insulin resistance and central (visceral) obesity play a pathogenic role [18,19], the clinical features are better defined [20–24], and the outcome is known. In fact, we have convincing evidence that the metabolic syndrome is a strong risk factor for T2DM and for cardiovascular disease (CVD). Despite this enormous progress in our knowledge of the syndrome, quite surprisingly we are now facing "the Metabolic Syndrome Paradox". The paradox consists in the fact that the syndrome is disputed now, when we know much, although not everything, about it and, in particular, just after the publication of dozens of papers focusing on the outcome. In the last year, in fact, the existence of the syndrome was challenged by Reaven, one of the pioneers in the field [20], who wrote a sort of obituitary on it, and by a group of experts appointed by the American Diabetes Association (ADA) and the European Association for the Study of Diabetes (EASD), who stated that the use of the term metabolic syndrome is misleading [21]. The concerns raised by the ADA-EASD experts can be summarized as follows: (1) diagnostic criteria are ambiguous and incomplete; (2) value of including diabetes in the definition is questionable; (3) insulin resistance as the unifying etiology is uncertain; (4) there is no clear basis for including/excluding other CVD risk factors; (5) CVD risk in subjects affected is variable and dependent on the specific risk factors present; (6) the CVD risk associated with the syndrome appears to be no greater than the sum of its parts; (7) treatment of the syndrome is not different from the treatment for each of its components; (8) the medical value of diagnosing the syndrome is unclear. Most of these concerns are justified, they must prompt to do more research and to look for more consensus, but, in my opinion they do not negate the existence of the metabolic syndrome. In this dispute, in fact, several virtues related to the "Metabolic Syndrome Approach" deserve to be mentioned.

3. The virtues of the "Metabolic Syndrome Approach"

Among the virtues of the "Metabolic Syndrome Approach" is that it prompts to seek carefully the other components when one is observed. In fact, isolated metabolic disorders are rare. In the Bruneck Study we observed that T2DM and the prediabetic conditions (impaired fasting glucose, IFG, and impaired glucose tolerance, IGT) occur very rarely as isolated conditions and even rarer was the finding of isolated hypertriglyceridemia or low HDL cholesterol [22]. In this study hypertension occurs 9-fold more frequently in association with other disorders than isolated [22]. In the same database, the cluster of 4 or 5 abnormalities in a given individual was 2 to 3-fold more frequent than expected by chance. This finding strongly supports the conclusion that one or more common denominators underlie the cluster. Among them, insulin resistance and central obesity are good candidates because both are associated, independently each other, with dysglycemia, dyslipidemia and hypertension, as well as intercorrelated [14].

In subjects with the metabolic syndrome the clinical phenotype can be fully blossomed, with all disorders well evident (e.g., T2DM), or partially expressed, with a cluster of mild to moderate abnormalities (e.g., IFG). Missing components or changes in the expression of components of the metabolic syndrome, however, should be carefully monitored over the

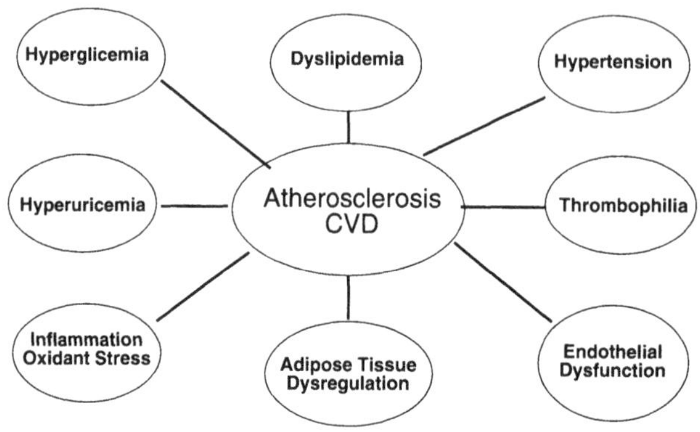

Fig. 2. The wide spectrum of pro-atherogenic disorders in the metabolic syndrome.

years. The clinical phenotype, indeed, is not static but rather dynamic and can evolve as a consequence of aging, changes in diet and/or physical activity, comorbidity and use of medications. A good example is T2DM. In the Bruneck Study we observed that the presence of the metabolic syndrome increased 4-fold the 10-year risk of T2DM in those without the disease at the baseline. However, when subjects without any metabolic disorder were the reference category, the risk of T2DM conveyed by a cluster of three disorders was 22-fold higher and the risk in those with 4–5 disorders was about 100-fold higher [Bonora et al, unpublished data]. This finding underscores the importance of using the appropriate reference category when estimating the risk.

The phenotype of the metabolic syndrome is not limited to central obesity, dyslipidemia, hypertension and dysglycemia, but often includes a variable array of abnormalities in coagulation, fibrinolysis, oxidant stress, innate immune response, adipocyte metabolic and endocrine activities, endothelial function. In fact, circulating levels of plasminogen activator inhibitor-1, fibrinogen, oxidized low density lipoproteins, C-reactive protein, white blood cells, ferritin, free fatty acids, leptin, and endothelial adhesion molecules (e.g., E-selectin or intracellular adhesion molecule-1) are generally higher in subjects with the metabolic syndrome [14,23–25]. On the other hand, adiponectin levels are generally lower in subjects with the syndrome who, therefore, have a wide spectrum of pro-atherogenic disorders (Fig. 2).

Another virtue of the “Metabolic Syndrome Approach” is that it emphasizes the high cardiovascular risk of subjects affected. Since its first descriptions in the literature it seemed that CVD could be a likely outcome in subjects with the metabolic syndrome. This hypothesis was recently confirmed by several longitudinal studies [26–38]. As shown in Table 1, which reports main results of some of these studies, the risk of coronary heart disease was 2- to 4-fold increased in subjects with the syndrome. Interestingly, the risk conveyed by the metabolic syndrome was greater in affected women than in affected men, and in subjects with pre-existing T2DM and/or CVD. In our experience, diabetic subjects with the metabolic syndrome had a 5-fold higher risk of CVD than subjects without the syndrome [39].

One of the concerns related to the metabolic syndrome is that the CVD risk is not substantially greater than the risk associated to diabetes or hypertension. However, this

Table 1
Risk of CHD morbidity or mortality in subjects with the metabolic syndrome

First author (study)	Country	No. of subjects	Years of follow-up	WHO criteria OR/HR/RR	NCEP criteria OR/HR/RR
Bonora (Bruneck Study)	Italy	888	5	2.03 (1.2–4.3)	1.50 (NS)
Isooma (Botnia Study)	Finland	3606	7	1.81 (1.24–2.65)	
Lakka (Kuopio Study)	Finland	1209	11	Men 2.87 (1.22–6.78)	Men 4.16 (1.60–10.8)
Sattar (WOSCOPS)	Scotland	6447	5		Men 1.30 (1.00–1.67)
Hu (DECODE)	Europe	11512	9	Men 2.26 (1.61–3.17) Women 2.78 (1.57–4.94)	
McNeill (ARIC)	USA	12089	11		Men 1.46 (1.23–1.74) Women 2.05 (1.59–2.64)
Hunt (SAHS)	USA	2815	13	Men 1.15 (NS) Women 2.83 (1.55–5.17)	Men 1.82 (1.14–2.91) Women 4.65 (2.35–9.21)
Malik (NHANES)	USA	6255	13		2.02 (1.42–2.89)

OR = odds ratio; HR = hazard ratio; RR = relative risk.
95% CI is given in parenthesis. See text for more details about the studies.

finding can be attributed to the use of subjects without the syndrome as reference category. Among these subjects, however, many have one or two metabolic abnormalities, including hypertension and/or T2DM, and this yielded an underestimation of the risk. In fact, when the reference category was composed of subjects without any metabolic disorder, the risk in subjects with the metabolic syndrome was definitely higher [29,33,35]. In the Bruneck Study this statistical approach allowed us to define a risk of CHD 6 to 12-fold higher in subjects with the metabolic syndrome than in individuals free of any metabolic abnormality, depending on the criteria used for diagnosing the syndrome [Bonora et al, unpublished data].

A further virtue of the "Metabolic Syndrome Approach" is that it draws attention to the cluster of "second line" risk factors, like IFG, IGT, large waist circumference, high triglycerides, low HDL cholesterol. These risk factors, when considered separately, are often neglected, but when they occur together in the same individuals the risk of CVD is very high. In the Bruneck Study the risk associated to the cluster of these "second line" risk factors could be appreciated only when the statistical approach was based upon considering them as part of the metabolic syndrome, and not when these traits were modelled separately [28]. In other words, one might underestimate the risk of CVD when these "second line" and often neglected risk factors are extrapolated by the clinical context.

4. Conclusions

The metabolic syndrome is a common condition in the general population. This condition is featured by the cluster of several traditional and non-traditional CVD risk factors. Affected subjects carry a very high risk of T2DM and CVD. The risk is particularly high if the appropriate reference category is used. If so, the risk of T2DM is about 20-fold higher and the risk of CVD is about 10-fold higher in subjects with the metabolic syndrome than in subjects without any metabolic disorder. The risk of CVD associated with the metabolic syndrome is higher in affected women that in affected men, and is particularly high when affected subjects have pre-existing T2DM and/or CVD. For such reasons the "Metabolic Syndrome Approach" is clinically useful in the definition of the risk. Moreover, the "Metabolic Syndrome Approach" draws attention to well defined underlying pathogenic factors of the cluster, i.e., central obesity and insulin resistance. These underlying factors can be targeted by specific interventions aiming at preventing the metabolic syndrome in those not affected yet, and T2DM and CVD in those already affected. Although many aspects related to the metabolic syndrome need to be better elucidated, and several concerns recently raised about the syndrome need to be adequately addressed by further investigations, the clinical value of identifying subjects with this common metabolic condition seems fully valid. The syndrome, therefore, is still alive. Long live the metabolic syndrome!

References

[1] E. Kylin, Studien ueber das Hypertonie–Hyperglykamie–Hyperurikamiesyndrom, Zentralblatt fuer Innere Medizin 44 (1923) 105–127.
[2] J. Vague, La differenciation sexuelle, factor determinants des formes de l'obesite, Press Med. 30 (1947) 339–340.
[3] P. Avogaro, et al., Associazione di iperlipemia, diabete mellito e obesità di medio grado, Acta Diabetol. Lat. 4 (1967) 572–590.
[4] G.M. Reaven, Banting lecture. Role of insulin resistance in human disease, Diabetes 37 (1988) 1595–1607.
[5] R.A. DeFronzo, E. Ferrannini, Insulin resistance: a multifaceted syndrome responsible for NIDDM, obesity, hypertension, dyslipidemia and atherosclerotic cardiovascular disease, Diabetes Care 14 (1991) 173–194.
[6] N.M. Kaplan, The deadly quartet: upper body obesity, glucose intolerance, hypertriglyceridemia and hypertension, Arch. Intern. Med. 149 (1989) 1514–1520.
[7] M. Modan, et al., A link between hypertension, obesity and glucose intolerance, J. Clin. Invest. 75 (1985) 809–817.
[8] I. Hjiermann, The metabolic cardiovascular syndrome: Syndrome X, Reaven's syndrome, insulin resistance syndrome, and atherothrombotic syndrome, J. Cardiovasc. Pharmacol. 20 (suppl 8) (1992) S5–S10.
[9] P.Z. Zimmet, Hyperinsulinemia. How innocent a bystander? Diabetes Care 16 (suppl 3) (1993) 56–70.
[10] WHO Consultation. Definition, diagnosis and classification of diabetes mellitus and its complications: Part 1. Diagnosis and classification of diabetes mellitus. World Health Organization, Geneva, Switzerland, 1999. Publication WHO/NCD/NCS/99.2.
[11] Expert Panel on Detection, Evaluation and Treatment of High Blood Cholesterol in Adults, Executive summary of the third report of the National Cholesterol Education Program (NCEP) Expert Panel on Detection, Evaluation and Treatment of High Blood Cholesterol in Adults (Adult Treatment Panel III), JAMA 285 (2001) 2486–2497.
[12] S.M. Grundy, et al., American Heart Association; National Heart, Lung, and Blood Institute. Diagnosis and management of the metabolic syndrome: an American Heart Association/National Heart, Lung, and Blood Institute Scientific Statement, Circulation 112 (2005) 2735–2752.
[13] K.G. Alberti, P. Zimmet, J. Shaw, Metabolic syndrome—a new world-wide definition. A Consensus Statement from the International Diabetes Federation, Diabet. Med. 23 (2006) 469–480.
[14] E. Bonora, et al., The metabolic syndrome: epidemiology and more extensive phenotypic description. Cross-sectional data from the Bruneck Study, Int. J. Obes. 27 (2003) 1283–1289.
[15] E.S. Ford, W. Giles, W.H. Dietz, Prevalence of the metabolic syndrome among US adults, JAMA 287 (2002) 356–359.
[16] J.B. Meigs, et al., Prevalence and characteristics of the metabolic syndrome in the San Antonio Heart and Framingham Offspring Studies, Diabetes 52 (2003) 2160–2167.
[17] B. Balkau, et al., European Group For The Study Of Insulin Resistance (EGIR). Frequency of the WHO metabolic syndrome in European cohorts, and al alternative definition of an insulin resistance syndrome, Diabetes Metab. 28 (2002) 364–376.

[18] R.H. Eckel, S.M. Grundy, P.Z. Zimmet, The metabolic syndrome, Lancet 365 (2005) 1415–1428.
[19] D.B. Carr, et al., Intra-abdominal fat is a major determinant of the National Cholesterol Education Program Adult Treatment Panel III criteria for the metabolic syndrome, Diabetes 53 (2004) 2087–2094.
[20] G.M. Reaven, The metabolic syndrome: requiescat in pace, Clin. Chem. 51 (2005) 931–938.
[21] R. Kahn, et al., The metabolic syndrome: time for a critical appraisal, Diabetes Care 28 (2005) 2289–2304.
[22] E. Bonora, et al., Prevalence of insulin resistance in metabolic disorders. The Bruneck Study, Diabetes 47 (1998) 1643–1649.
[23] I. Toft, et al., Gender differences in the relationships between plasma plasminogen activator inhibitor-1 activity and factors linked to the insulin resistance syndrome in essential hypertension, Arterioscler. Thromb. Vasc. Biol. 17 (1997) 553–559.
[24] G. Imperatore, et al., Plasma fibrinogen: a new factor of the metabolic syndrome, Diabetes Care 21 (1998) 649–654 CRP.
[25] A. Festa, et al., Chronic subclinical inflammation as part of the insulin resistance syndrome. The Insulin Resistance Atherosclerosis Study (IRAS), Circulation 102 (2000) 42–47.
[26] B. Isomaa, et al., Cardiovascular morbidity and mortality associated with metabolic syndrome, Diabetes Care 24 (2001) 683–689.
[27] H.M. Lakka, The metabolic syndrome and total and cardiovascular disease mortality in middle-aged men, JAMA 288 (2002) 2709–2716.
[28] E. Bonora, et al., Carotid atherosclerosis and coronary heart disease in the metabolic syndrome. Prospective data from the Bruneck Study, Diabetes Care 26 (2003) 1251–1257.
[29] N. Sattar, et al., Metabolic syndrome with and without C-reactive protein as a predictor of coronary heart disease and diabetes in the west of Scotland coronary prevention study, Circulation 108 (2003) 414–419.
[30] P.M. Ridker, et al., C-reactive protein, the metabolic syndrome, and risk of incident cardiovascular events. An 8-year follow-up of 14719 initially healthy American women, Circulation 107 (2003) 391–397.
[31] G. Hu, et al., for the DECODE Study Group. Prevalence of the metabolic syndrome and its relation to all-cause and cardiovascular mortality in nondiabetic european men and women, Arch. Intern. Med. 164 (2004) 1066–1076.
[32] K.J. Hunt, et al., National cholesterol education program versus World Health Organization metabolic syndrome in relation to all-cause and cardiovascular mortality in the San Antonio Heart Study, Circulation 110 (2004) 1251–1257.
[33] S. Malik, et al., Impact of the metabolic syndrome on mortality from coronary heart disease, cardiovascular disease, and all causes in United States adults, Circulation 110 (2004) 1245–1250.
[34] C.J. Girman, et al., 4S Group and the AFCAPS/TexCAPS Research Group. The metabolic syndrome and risk of major coronary events in the Scandinavian Simvastatin Survival Study (4S) and the Air Force/Texas Coronary Atherosclerosis Prevention Study (AFCAPS/TexCAPS), Am. J. Cardiol. 93 (2004) 136–141.
[35] A. McNeill, et al., The metabolic syndrome and 11-year risk of incident cardiovascular disease in the Atherosclerosis Risk in Communities Study, Diabetes Care 28 (2005) 385–390.
[36] M.K. Rutter, et al., C-reactive protein, the metabolic syndrome and prediction of cardiovascular events in the Framingham Offspring Study, Circulation 110 (2004) 380–385.
[37] A. Scuteri, et al., Cardiovascular Health Study. The metabolic syndrome in older individuals: prevalence and prediction of cardiovascular events: the Cardiovascular Health Study, Diabetes Care 28 (2005) 882–887.
[38] J.M. Dekker, et al., Metabolic syndrome and 10-year cardiovascular disease risk in the Hoorn Study, Circulation 112 (2005) 666–673.
[39] E. Bonora, et al., The metabolic syndrome is an independent predictor of cardiovascular disease in type 2 diabetic subjects. Prospective data from the Verona Diabetes Complications Study, Diabet. Med. 21 (2004) 52–58.

ELSEVIER

International Congress Series 1303 (2007) 10–20

www.ics-elsevier.com

Global management of high risk patients: Integrated primary cardiovascular prevention in diabetics

Andrea A. Conti [a,b,c,*], Martina Minelli [a], Gian Franco Gensini [a,b,c]

[a] *Dipartimento di Area Critica Medico Chirurgica, Università degli Studi di Firenze, Italy*
[b] *Fondazione Don Carlo Gnocchi, IRCCS Firenze, Italy*
[c] *Centro Italiano per la Medicina Basata sulle Prove, Firenze, Italy*

Abstract. Diabetes mellitus is a pivotal risk factor for cardiovascular disease and a negative prognostic element in cardiovascular patients. The incidence of cardiovascular diseases in diabetics is 3-to-6 times higher than in non-diabetics, and cardiovascular pathology progresses more quickly in the former, thus constituting their major determinant of mortality. In diabetics 65–75% of deaths are caused by cardiovascular factors, and following a major coronary event diabetes increases about 2–3 times the all-cause mortality risk in affected people. Diabetes is also associated with a triple risk of death from coronary heart disease and a 10–12-fold increase in risk of mortality from coronary heart disease if compared with people with neither diabetes mellitus nor coronary heart disease. A healthy lifestyle, including cessation of smoking, suitable exercise, correct diet, appropriate weight loss and stress control, should be recommended to every subject in the perspective of cardiovascular prevention. Additional specific recommendations for diabetics in the primary prevention of cardiovascular events include accurate individually tailored glycemic control (general target: HbA1c < 7%), strict blood pressure treatment (target: < 130/80 mmHg), optimal lipid lowering regimen (target: LDL-C < 100 mg/dl; < 70 mg/dl in very high risk diabetics), antiplatelet therapy with aspirin (dosage: 75–150 mg per day). The current and future objective for health operators and systems is that of harmonically integrating multiple risk factor management not only with stringent treatment goals, but also with selective attention to the specific needs and fundamental values of every diabetic person encountered in daily clinical practice.

Keywords: Diabetes mellitus; Cardiovascular disease; Prevention; Risk factors; Evidence-based medicine; Clinical guidelines; History of medicine

* Corresponding author. Dipartimento di Area Critica Medico Chirurgica, Università degli Studi di Firenze, Viale Morgagni 85, I-50134, Firenze, Italy. Tel.: +39 055 417928; fax: +39 055 4379384.
E-mail address: aa.conti@dac.unifi.it (A.A. Conti).

0531-5131/ © 2007 Published by Elsevier B.V.
doi:10.1016/j.ics.2007.03.028

1. The concept of risk through time

Accurate risk assessment is one of the major challenges of current clinical medicine. The definition of risk appears to be variable through different settings and different times, but in the cardiovascular context by risk is now generally meant the probability of developing a clinical event through time estimated on the basis of the quantification of the presence, and, if feasible, of the interaction, of different pathologies and/or risk factors [1].

The modern concept of risk factor in the biomedical field is quite a recent methodological achievement, since in the past it was the concept of direct ("infectious" like) causality that prevailed [2]. Causal criteria oriented in an inductive way go back to the eighteenth century, as in the indications given by David Hume (1711–1776) [3]. Such criteria were used to develop inferences useful in distinguishing causal from non-causal determinants, and the inductive canons of John Stuart Mill (1806–1873), formulated in the nineteenth century, represent a good historical example of this [4]. A major epistemological problem with nineteenth century biomedicine, however, was the fact that the predominance of acute, or sub-acute, mono-causal diseases (such as the infectious ones), led researchers of that time to privilege the fallacious perspective that a single, sufficient and necessary causative agent could be identified in virtually every disease [1].

The epidemiological transition typical of the twentieth century, the historical period in which, at least in the Western World, quick onset and rapidly evolving mono-factorial pathologies have ceded the epidemiological field to multi-factorial, chronically degenerative, typically slowly evolving diseases, has determined the awareness that a rigid causal model could no longer be sufficient to understand largely diffused diseases [5]. Cardiovascular and neoplastic disorders have, in the course of the last sixty years, prompted the need to define their "risk factors", meaning those elements predisposing to, and/or increasing the risk of, the development of multi-factorial chronic pathologies. In the second half of the twentieth century, therefore, deterministic biomedical patterns were flanked and superseded by probabilistic considerations regarding the insurgence and evolution of pathologic phenomena [6].

In the epidemiological field much of the merit of this paradigm modification must be ascribed to Sir Austin Bradford Hill (1897–1991), who accurately defined the causal criteria in epidemiology [7]. Far from being mechanical determinants for the identification of the direct cause of diseases, these criteria were formulated, in the biological scenario, to identify the features of the epidemiological association functional in defining the causal, the predisposing and the risk-increasing elements involved in the insurgence and in the development of a disease. In synthesis, a set of epidemiological–methodological criteria are to be contemporaneously present in order to characterize a "real" risk factor as such, namely the now classical dimensions of specificity, consistency, coherence, strength, temporality, biologic gradient, experimental evidence and plausibility. Although this last dimension is still today much debated (essentially because the current plausibility of matters depends on current knowledge, and if and when such knowledge is limited, it fallaciously prevents the establishment of plausibility, even when the latter would be possible), general consensus has now been attained for the other criteria in correctly defining risk factors [8].

Appropriate analytical studies can today provide estimates for the "attributable risk", useful in measuring the role of exposure in the determination of a pathological picture, and subsequently in quantifying the "preventable fraction" of the same disease, that is, the effect obtainable when deleting or controlling the associated exposure [1]. It is now well known that the attributable risk and the preventable fraction of diabetes mellitus dependent cardiovascular disease may be accurately estimated and are definitely high; in effect, besides being a full disease per se, diabetes is currently considered a well established risk factor (some authors already define it as a "classical" risk factor) for cardiovascular diseases [9]. Diabetes is also a negative prognostic pathological element placing cardiovascular patients at a consistently higher risk of major clinical events, and therefore its primary (before its insurgence) and its secondary (the prophylaxis of its consequences in diabetic individuals) prevention should be strongly recommended and widely implemented. In turn, cardiovascular prevention of diabetic patients (who, by definition, are high risk patients) with unknown cardiovascular diseases must also be carefully carried out (i.e. the cardiovascular primary prevention of diabetic subjects, as understood in this contribution). The description of the optimal current cardiovascular management of this last category of high risk patients is the primary objective of this paper.

2. Diabetes mellitus and cardiovascular diseases

The complete definition of diabetes mellitus includes a set of disorders characterized by chronic hyperglycemia as a result of (usually) multiple defects in insulin secretion and/or action, which give rise to concomitant modifications of the human metabolism of carbohydrates, proteins and fats [10]. Diabetes is currently considered as the clinical result of a progressive qualitative and quantitative disturbance of glucose metabolism whose numerical humoral definition foresees a fasting venous glucose of at least 7 mmol/l or a plasma venous glucose of at least 11.1 mmol/l two hours after an oral glucose load of 75 mg, on two or more occasions [11].

This operational definition of diabetes mellitus is essential in distinguishing diabetes mellitus within the large spectrum of glucose metabolism disorders, which include impaired glucose tolerance, defined when fasting venous glucose is less than 7 mmol/l or at least 7.8 mmol/l two hours after 75 g oral glucose load, and also impaired fasting glycemia, namely the presence of fasting venous glucose included between 6.1 and 7 mmol/l.

Type I diabetes is the clinical and humoral picture of diabetes mellitus in the case in which the endocrine pancreas synthesizes and releases too little insulin, if none at all, because of the massive destruction of its beta cells. Type II diabetes is in turn the clinical and humoral result of concomitant multiple defects in insulin secretion and action, and its incidence increases with increasing age and decreasing physical activity. Type II diabetes is more frequent in subjects affected by dyslipidemia, hypertension and obesity, which are well known cardiovascular risk factors [12].

The connections of diabetes mellitus with cardiovascular diseases are numerous and close. In effect, not only are the links between diabetes and the other risk factors multiple (e.g. hypertension is 2–3 times more prevalent in diabetics than in non-diabetics), but also the direct relationships between already diagnosed cardiovascular pathology, in particular coronary heart disease, and diabetes mellitus are well established and notable [13].

Coronary heart disease is a major determinant of mortality and morbidity in the whole world, since it accounts alone for more than 12% of deaths and for a heavy burden of disability [14]. The biggest proportion of this burden may be ascribed to a number of classical risk factors for cardiovascular disease, including also diabetes mellitus, whose negative role in the prognosis of cardiovascular pathology is becoming more and more relevant [15]. The incidence of cardiovascular diseases in diabetic people is 3-to-6 times more frequent if compared to non-diabetics. Almost 50% of middle aged and older Caucasian subjects with diabetes mellitus have documented evidence of coronary artery disease, approximately twice that of non-diabetic individuals extracted from the same population. Moreover, cardiovascular pathology progresses more quickly in diabetics than in non-diabetics, thus constituting the major determinant of mortality in these patients, in whom 65–75% of deaths are caused by cardiovascular causes (in particular, in more than 50% of the cases, coronary heart disease). Following a major coronary event diabetes mellitus augments the mortality risk in affected people of around 2–3 times [16]. Overall, diabetes per se is associated with a double risk of all-cause mortality, a triple risk of death from coronary heart disease and a 10–12-fold increase in risk of mortality from coronary heart disease if compared with people with neither diabetes mellitus nor coronary heart disease [17]. These impressive data make clear why the "cardiovascular" prevention of high risk patients, such as diabetic ones, is so urgent in the current clinical and epidemiological world scenario, characterized by an epidemic of diabetes and, even worse, of "diabesity", that is, the negative combination of diabetes mellitus and obesity [18].

3. Integrated clinical cardiovascular prevention in diabetic patients: from research evidence to clinical recommendations

A healthy lifestyle, including cessation of smoking, suitable exercise, correct diet, appropriate weight and stress control, should be recommended to every subject in the perspective of cardiovascular prevention [19]. Additional specific recommendations for diabetic patients derive from currently available clinical evidence (Fig. 1) [20].

3.1. Glycemic control

In the nineties the role of intensive glycemic control was proposed as crucial in diabetic patients, especially in the perspective of cardiovascular prevention [21]. Aggressive strategies proved to be of benefit in type I diabetic patients, if compared to conventional control, as evidenced in a systematic review demonstrating that intensive control adopted for more than two years was able to reduce the frequency of a first major clinical cardiovascular event in type I diabetic subjects [22,23]. The cardiovascular preventive picture is less clear in people with type II diabetes mellitus, since controlled clinical studies, while evidencing a higher number of hypoglycemic episodes and of cases of weight increase in diabetics undergoing intensive glycemic control, could not always document significant differences in cardiovascular mortality and morbidity between intensive and conventional glycemic control strategies [24,25]. However, systematic reviews indicate that, compared to standard care, intensive glycemic control programmes can reduce in a significant way, over periods included between 3 and 4 years, HbA1c percentage in type II diabetic patients, thus nearing the HbA1c target currently considered the golden standard for diabetics in the primary prevention of cardiovascular disease [26].

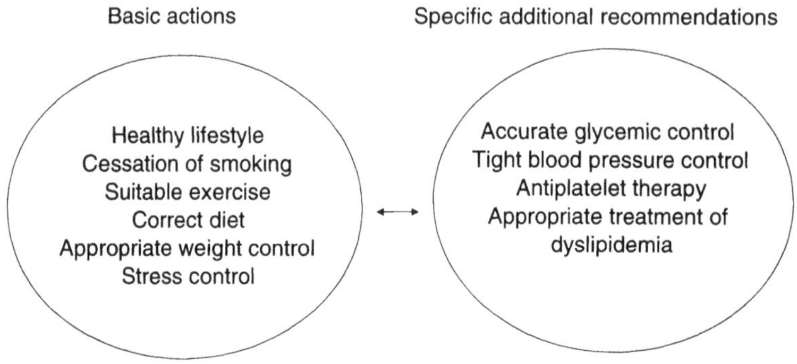

Fig. 1. Evidence-based interventions for integrated clinical cardiovascular prevention in diabetic patients.

The Numbers Needed to Treat (NNTs) in relevant studies regarding the primary prevention of cardiovascular events in diabetics with specific reference to glycemic control may be summarised as follows:

UKPDS (Intensive treatment with metformin versus conventional regimen) 16 (10–71);
UKPDS (Intensive treatment with insulin and/or sulphonylurea versus conventional regimen) 46;
DCCT (Type I diabetes) 45 (28–728) [11].

3.2. Blood pressure control

Clinical and epidemiological evidence clearly indicates that, if compared with no anti-hypertensive therapy, blood pressure control in hypertensive diabetics significantly reduces cardiovascular morbidity and mortality. Moreover, blood pressure lowering to diastolic values of 80 mmHg or less reduces to a higher extent the occurrence of major clinical cardiovascular events [27]. To achieve such objectives, different pharmacological classes of antihypertensive drugs have been widely investigated in clinical trials, namely diuretics, calcium channel blockers, beta blockers, angiotensin converting enzyme inhibitors and angiotensin II receptor antagonists [28]. They have all proved to be effective in reducing mortality and morbidity in hypertensive diabetics, particularly in elderly people [29]. Ramipril reduces in a significant way not only the occurrence of cardiovascular events, but also the progression rate of nephropathy in diabetic subjects, if compared to placebo, and the use of ramipril in addition to other therapies should therefore be recommended in diabetics with dyslipidemia or other cardiovascular risk factors [30]. Patients on beta blockers (atenolol), compared to ACE-inhibitor therapy (captopril), have increased to a higher extent their body weight in randomised controlled studies, although no significant difference between the two classes of drugs has emerged with regard to cardiovascular events [31,32]. Subjects on atenolol have shown a higher degree of withdrawal from therapy when compared with hypertensive diabetics on angiotensin II receptor antagonists (losartan). The same losartan has reduced cardiovascular events, as compared to atenolol, in diabetic people with hypertension and left ventricular hypertrophy. Losartan and irbesartan have recently been shown to determine renal protection similar to that of ACE-inhibitors in diabetics with hypertension and/or left ventricular hypertrophy [33–36].

Table 1
Numbers Needed To Treat (with their 95% confidence intervals) in relevant studies regarding the primary prevention of cardiovascular events in diabetics with specific reference to blood pressure control (11 modified)

Trial	Reference	NNT(95% CI)
ABCD	Estacio RO, et al. [40] N Engl J Med 1998; 338: 645–52	12 (10–19)
Syst-Eur	Tuomilehto J, et al. [38] N Engl J Med 1999; 340: 677–84	13 (10–31)
UKPDS	UKPDS Group. [31] BMJ 1998; 317: 703–13	14 (9–35) (myocardial infarction).
FACET	Tatti P, et al. [39] Diabetes Care 1998; 21: 597–603	15 (10–199)
	Berl T, et al. [52] Ann Intern Med 2003; 138: 542–549	15
HOT	Hansson L, et al. [27] Lancet 1998; 351: 1751–62	22 (16–57)

Diuretic chlorthalidone has proved to be as effective as the ACE-inhibitor lisinopril in reducing clinical vascular events in an ample randomised clinical trial [37]. This same diuretic agent has proved to be not inferior to calcium channel blocker amlodipine in reducing cardiovascular clinical episodes in diabetic people, while reducing heart failure if compared to that same calcium channel blocker [38]. The ACE-inhibitors enalapril and fosinopril have significantly reduced cardiovascular events in randomised controlled trials comparing them with the calcium channel blockers nisoldipine and amlodipine [39–41].

The NNTs in relevant studies regarding the primary prevention of cardiovascular events in diabetics with specific reference to blood pressure control are summarised in Table 1 [11].

3.3. Antiplatelet therapy

Clinical evidence regarding the secondary prevention potential of aspirin in cardiovascular diseases is clear and convincing: methodologically sound systematic reviews indicate that aspirin, compared to placebo, reduces the incidence of major cardiovascular events and even mortality from any cause in cardiovascular patients [42]. Data on aspirin treatment in diabetics without diagnosed cardiovascular disease (primary prevention) are not fully coherent, since randomised controlled trials have shown that aspirin, compared to placebo, can reduce the risk of acute myocardial infarction in the course of five years, while other clinical trials have not found any statistically significant cardiovascular benefit from antiplatelet therapy in diabetics [43]. However, since diabetics over 40 years or with additional cardiovascular risk factors must be considered at increased risk, aspirin in the prevention of cardiovascular events in these diabetics should therefore be suggested, as emphasised by the most recent clinical practice guidelines for cardiovascular prevention [20] on the basis of methodologically robust clinical trials [27,44,45].

The NNTs in relevant studies regarding the primary prevention of cardiovascular events in diabetics with specific reference to aspirin therapy may be summarised as follows:

Physician's Health Study 16 (12–47);
ETDRS 39 (21–716) [11].

3.4. Treatment of dyslipidemia

Statins are effective and safe drugs for cardiovascular disease management [46]. A large amount of data indicates that they significantly reduce the incidence of major cardiovascular

Table 2
Numbers Needed To Treat (with their 95% confidence intervals) in relevant studies regarding the primary prevention of cardiovascular events in diabetics with specific reference to the treatment of dyslipidemia (11 modified)

Trial	Reference	NNT (95%CI)
SENDCAP	Elkeles RS, et al. [49] Diabetes Care 1998; 21: 641–8	6 (5–20)
HPS	HPS Collaborative Group. [48] Lancet 2003;361:2005–16	20 (13–28)
AFCAPS/TexCAPS	Downs JR, et al. [47] JAMA 1998; 279: 1615–22	27

events if compared to placebo, and clinical evidence demonstrates that statins improve in a coherent way different cardiovascular end points in diabetic people. With regard to the appropriate intensity of lipid lowering therapy in diabetes, intervention studies have demonstrated that aggressive lipid lowering (atorvastatin for a LDL target of less than 100 mg/dl) can reduce to a higher extent cardiovascular mortality and morbidity as compared with a standard dyslipidemia treatment [47]. Simvastatin 40 mg per day has proved to be able to reduce significantly the incidence of major cardiovascular events in diabetics with a total cholesterol value higher than 3.5 mmol/l, as demonstrated by the Heart Protection Study [48]. Fibrates have also proved effective in reducing the incidence of cardiovascular clinical events if compared to placebo [49]. Statins are however currently considered the gold standard for lipid lowering in hypertensive diabetics [29,50,51]. Newly formulated combinations, such as the promising association of statin with ezetimibe, which, if compared to statin alone, has already proved to be effective in reducing LDL-C in diabetic subjects already in therapy with statins, need further research.

The NNTs in relevant studies regarding the primary prevention of cardiovascular events in diabetics with specific reference to the treatment of dyslipidemia are summarised in Table 2 [11].

Shifting from the best biomedical evidence to the optimal clinical recommendations, the following indications emerge from the most updated guidelines on cardiovascular prevention in diabetic individuals without known cardiovascular disease [20]. Individually tailored accurate glycemic control with exercise, diet and hypoglycemic oral drugs or insulin is a cornerstone in the management of every diabetic subject, particularly in the perspective of primary cardiovascular prevention (target: HbA1c < 7%). Strict blood pressure control is essential in diabetics (target blood pressure:< 130/80 mmHg); ACE inhibitors, thiazide diuretics, calcium channel blockers, beta blockers and angiotensin II receptor antagonists have all proved to be effective agents. An adapted choice of molecules, combinations and dosages is indicated in accordance with the individual clinical profile; multiple-drug therapy is usually necessary to obtain blood pressure targets. Since ACE inhibitors have been proved to play a major role in renal protection in diabetic hypertensive people, current clinical views point to the fact that ramipril, for its global protective effect (including renal benefit) should be recommended in addition to other therapies in diabetics with dyslipidemia or other cardiovascular risk factors such as hypertension. Recently angiotensin II receptor antagonists (losartan, irbesartan) have also proved to have a similar beneficial impact on the kidney, in particular in subjects with left ventricular hypertrophy [52]. Therefore, patients with diabetes and hypertension should be treated with a therapy including either an ACE inhibitor or an angiotensin II receptor antagonist; beta blockers, thiazide diuretics or calcium channel blockers should be added as appropriate to obtain blood pressure targets. Statins are the gold standard for hypercholesterolemia management in diabetic patients. In high risk patients, such as diabetics, the currently recommended LDL-C goal is <100 mg/dl, and a LDL-C goal <70 mg/dl is a therapeutic option in patients considered at very high risk (e.g. diabetics with multiple cardiovascular risk factors, even in the absence of known cardiovascular disease). Statins and fibrates may both be required when managing combined hyperlipidemia. The recent promising results of the pharmacological association of a statin with ezetimibe represent important clinical achievements that need to be confirmed in very large populations of diabetic people. In general, aspirin 75–150 mg should be recommended for all diabetic patients at increased cardiovascular risk, including individuals over 40 years or carrying additional risk factors; given that diabetes must be considered a risk equivalent of coronary heart disease, aspirin in the prevention of cardiovascular events in diabetic people should therefore be suggested as indicated above, provided that major contraindications for its use are ruled out and that blood pressure is controlled to minimise the risk of hemorrhagic stroke [20].

4. Concluding remarks

Isolated treatment of different risk factors for cardiovascular disease in diabetic subjects has already proved to be substantially effective and safe in controlled settings. However, current and future objectives for health professionals and systems are those of integrating multiple risk factor management with stringent treatment goals in the real world. Existing clinical evidence indicates that the intensive management of concomitant risk factors in type II diabetic people is feasible and effective, as documented by randomised trials showing a reduction in major cardiovascular events in the course of eight years by treating diabetics with an integrated aggressive approach, as compared to a standard therapy according to clinical guidelines [29]. Health operators should therefore be fully aware of the challenging objective awaiting them and their diabetic patients in sharing optimal complete management of diabetes mellitus in a cardiovascular prevention perspective.

In effect, as is well shown by intense glycemia control programmes, these are really and effectively implemented if the degree of motivation and of education of participants is high. Such elevated levels may be difficult to achieve outside controlled settings, such as those of randomised clinical trials, but it is exactly outside them, in the real world, that the vast majority of health professionals are called upon to reach the best concordance with diabetic patients.

If it is true that the global management of diabetic patients in the ample perspective of integrated cardiovascular prevention must be based on the best research evidence giving rise to applicable clinical recommendations, such as the ones synthesized in this paper, it is even more true that the actual implementation of these recommendations cannot do without individually tailored attention to the specific preferences, the general needs and the fundamental values of each and every diabetic person encountered in daily clinical practice.

Acknowledgements

The authors would like to thank Professor Luisa Camaiora, B.A., M.Phil., for her correction of the English.

References

[1] K.J. Rothman, S. Greenland, Modern Epidemiology, 2nd edition, Lippincott-Raven Publishers, Philadelphia, PA, USA, 1998.
[2] K.J. Rothman (Ed.), Causal Inference, Epidemiology Resources, Boston, 1988.
[3] Hume D. A treatise of human nature. Oxford: Oxford University Press, 1888; 2nd edition, 1978 (original publication, 1739).
[4] J.S.A. Mill, System of Logic, Ratiocinative and Inductive, 5th edition, Parker, Son and Bowin, London, 1862.
[5] G.F. Gensini, A.A. Conti, D. Lippi, Evolution of the epidemiologic context of cardiovascular diseases: a critical historical approach, Ital. Heart J 3 (Suppl 6) (2002) 5S–8S.
[6] A.A. Conti, C. Galanti, G.F. Gensini, Is evidence-based medicine really a craze? Surely it is fashionable to criticize it. A methodologic comment from the Centro Italiano per la Medicina Basata sulle Prove (Italian Center for Evidence-Based Medicine), Ital. Heart J Suppl 1 (2000) 1192–1195.
[7] A.B. Hill, The environment and disease: association or causation? Proc. R. Soc. Med. 58 (1965) 295–300.
[8] D.L. Weed, On the logic of causal inference, Am. J. Epidemiol. 123 (1986) 965–979.
[9] MJ. Harris (Ed.), Diabetes in America, 2nd edition, National Institutes of Health, Bethesda, MD, 1995.
[10] K. Alberti, P. Zimmet, Definition, diagnosis and classification of diabetes mellitus and its complications. Part 1: diagnosis and classification of diabetes mellitus. Provisional report of a WHO consultation, Diabet. Med. 15 (1998) 539–553.
[11] BMJ Clinical Evidence Online, BMJ Publishing Group, London, UK; available online at: http://www.clinicalevidence.com/ceweb/products/online_only.jsp (accessed on April 13th, 2007).
[12] A.S. Krolewski, J.H. Warram, M.B. Freire, Epidemiology of late diabetic complications. A basis for the development and evaluation of preventive programs, Endocrinol. Metab. Clin. N. Am. 25 (1996) 217–242.
[13] S.M. Haffner, et al., Metabolic syndrome, new onset diabetes and new end points in cardiovascular trials, J. Cardiovasc. Pharmacol. 47 (2006) 469–475.
[14] E. Braunwald, A.S. Fauci, D.L. Kasper, S.L. Hauser, D.L. Longo, J.L. Jameson (Eds.), Harrison's Principles of Internal Medicine, 15th edition, McGraw-Hill, New York, 2001.
[15] S.F. Dinneen, H.C. Gerstein, The association of microalbuminuria and mortality in non-insulin-dependent diabetes mellitus: a systematic overview of the literature, Arch. Intern. Med. 157 (1997) 1413–1438.
[16] L. Goldman, D. Ausiello (Eds.), Cecil Textbook of Medicine, 22nd edition, Saunders, Philadelphia, 2004.
[17] D.J. Weatherall, T.M. Cox, J.D. Firth, E.J. Benz (Eds.), Oxford Textbook of Medicine, 4th edition, Oxford Medical Publications, Oxford, 2003.
[18] K. Suastika, Update in the management of obesity, Acta Med. Indones. 38 (2006) 231–237.
[19] D. Wood, et al., Clinicians' manual on total risk management, in: L. Davenport (Ed.), A Guide to Prevention of Coronary Heart Disease, Science Press, London, 2000.
[20] J.B. Buse, et al., Primary prevention of cardiovascular diseases in people with diabetes mellitus. A scientific statement from the American Heart Association and the American Diabetes Association, Circulation 115 (2007) 114–126.
[21] Y. Groeneveld, et al., Relationship between blood glucose level and mortality in type 2 diabetes mellitus: a systematic review, Diabet. Med. 16 (1999) 2–13.
[22] DCCT Research Group, The effect of intensive treatment of diabetes on the development and progression of long-term complications in insulin-dependent diabetes mellitus, N. Engl. J. Med. 329 (1993) 977–986.
[23] DCCT Research Group, Effect of intensive diabetes management on macrovascular events and risk factors in the Diabetes Control and Complications Trial, Am. J. Cardiol. 75 (1995) 894–903.
[24] UK Prospective Diabetes Study Group, Intensive blood-glucose control with sulphonylureas or insulin compared with conventional treatment and risk of complications in patients with type 2 diabetes. UKPDS 33, Lancet 352 (1998) 837–853.
[25] UK Prospective Diabetes Study Group, Effect of intensive blood-glucose control with metformin on complications in overweight patients with type 2 diabetes. UKPDS 34, Lancet 352 (1998) 854–865.
[26] A.R. Vasudevan, C.M. Ballantyne, Cardiometabolic risk assessment: an approach to the prevention of cardiovascular disease and diabetes mellitus, Clin. Cornerstone 7 (2005) 7–16.
[27] L. Hansson, et al., Effects of intensive blood-pressure lowering and low-dose aspirin in patients with hypertension: principal results of the Hypertension Optimal Treatment (HOT) randomised trial, Lancet 351 (1998) 1751–1762.

[28] J. Fuller, et al., Antihypertensive therapy for preventing cardiovascular complications in people with diabetes, Cochrane Database Syst. Rev. 1 (2003) CD002188.
[29] The practical implementation taskforce for the prevention of cardiovascular disease. Prevention of cardiovascular disease: an evidence-based clinical aid 2004, MJA Focus, vol. 181, 2004, pp. F1–F14.
[30] Heart Outcomes Prevention Evaluation (HOPE) Study Investigators, Effects of ramipril on cardiovascular and microvascular outcomes in people with diabetes mellitus: results of the HOPE study and the MICRO-HOPE substudy, Lancet 355 (2000) 253–259.
[31] UK Prospective Diabetes Study Group, Tight blood pressure control and risk of macrovascular complications in type 2 diabetes. UKPDS 38, BMJ 317 (1998) 703–713.
[32] UK Prospective Diabetes Study Group, Efficacy of atenolol and captopril in reducing risk of macrovascular and microvascular complications in type 2 diabetes. UKPDS 39, BMJ 317 (1998) 713–720.
[33] E. Lewis, et al., Renoprotective effect of the angiotensin-receptor antagonist irbesartan in patients with nephropathy due to type 2 diabetes, N. Engl. J. Med. 345 (2001) 851–860.
[34] H. Parving, et al., The effect of irbesartan on the development of diabetic nephropathy in patients with type 2 diabetes, N. Engl. J. Med. 345 (2001) 870–878.
[35] B. Brenner, et al., Effect of losartan on renal and cardiovascular outcomes in patients with type 2 diabetes and nephropathy, N. Engl. J. Med. 345 (2001) 861–869.
[36] L. Lindholm, et al., Cardiovascular morbidity and mortality in patients with diabetes in the Losartan Intervention For Endpoint reduction in hypertension study (LIFE): a randomised trial against atenolol, Lancet 359 (2002) 1004–1010.
[37] ALLHAT Collaborative Research Group, Major cardiovascular events in hypertensive patients randomised to doxazosin vs chlorthalidone: the antihypertensive and lipid-lowering treatment to prevent heart attack trial (ALLHAT), JAMA 283 (2000) 1967–1975.
[38] J. Tuomilehto, et al., Effects of calcium-channel blockade in older patients with diabetes and systolic hypertension, N. Engl. J. Med. 340 (1999) 677–684.
[39] P. Tatti, et al., Outcome results of the fosinopril versus amlodipine cardiovascular events randomised trial (FACET) in patients with hypertension and NIDDM, Diabetes Care 21 (1998) 597–603.
[40] R.O. Estacio, et al., The effect of nisoldipine as compared with enalapril on cardiovascular events in patients with NIDDM and hypertension, N. Engl. J. Med. 338 (1998) 645–652.
[41] L. Hansson, et al., Effect of angiotensin-converting enzyme inhibition compared with conventional therapy on cardiovascular morbidity and mortality in hypertension. The Captopril Prevention Project (CAPPP) randomised trial, Lancet 353 (1999) 611–616.
[42] C. Nobles-James, E.A. James, J.R. Sowers, Prevention of cardiovascular complications of diabetes mellitus by aspirin, Cardiovasc. Drug Rev. 22 (2004) 215–226.
[43] ETDRS Investigators, Aspirin effects on mortality and morbidity in patients with diabetes mellitus, JAMA 268 (1992) 1292–1300.
[44] Steering Committee of the Physicians' Health Study Research Group, Final report on the aspirin component of the ongoing Physicians' Health Study, N. Engl. J. Med. 321 (1989) 129–135.
[45] Collaborative overview of randomised trials of antiplatelet therapy I: prevention of death, myocardial infarction and stroke by prolonged antiplatelet therapy in various categories of patients. Antiplatelet Trialists' Collaboration (ATC), BMJ 308 (1994) 81–106.
[46] R.M. Guthrie, Rising to the challenge of treating high-risk patients, Am. J. Manag. Care 12 (2006) S318–S324.
[47] J.R. Downs, et al., Primary prevention of acute coronary events with lovastatin in men and women with average cholesterol levels: results of AFCAPS/TexCAPS. Air Force/Texas Coronary Atherosclerosis Prevention Study, JAMA 279 (1998) 1615–1622.
[48] Heart Protection Study Collaborative Group, MRC/BHF heart protection study of cholesterol-lowering with simvastatin in 5963 people with diabetes: a randomised placebo-controlled trial, Lancet 361 (2003) 2005–2016.
[49] R.S. Elkeles, et al., Cardiovascular outcomes in type 2 diabetes. A double-blind placebo-controlled study of bezafibrate: the St Mary's, Ealing, Northwick Park Diabetes Cardiovascular Disease Prevention (SENDCAP) Study, Diabetes Care 21 (1998) 641–648.
[50] P. Koskinen, et al., Coronary heart disease incidence in NIDDM patients in the Helsinki Heart Study, Diabetes Care 15 (1992) 820–825.

[51] G.F. Gensini, A.A. Conti, Evidence-based evaluation of benefits in therapeutic interventions: methodologically controlled and non-randomly assigned reflections on the number needed to treat, Ital. Heart J 4 (2003) 80–83.
[52] T. Berl, et al., Cardiovascular outcomes in the Irbesartan Diabetic Nephropathy Trial of patients with type 2 diabetes and overt nephropathy, Ann. Intern. Med. 138 (2003) 542–549.

The Metabolic Syndrome: a widespread inflammatory disease

International Congress Series 1303 (2007) 23–30

ELSEVIER

www.ics-elsevier.com

Inflammation and macrophage infiltration in adipose tissue: A link between diabetes and atherosclerosis

Rossella Menghini, Renato Lauro, Massimo Federici *

Department of Internal Medicine, University of Rome Tor Vergata, Rome, Italy

Abstract. Obesity is associated with macrophage infiltration of adipose tissue, resulting in the development of insulin resistance and cardiovascular diseases. MCP-1 is involved in monocyte recruitment to both early atherosclerotic lesion and adipose tissue. We recently described two possible mechanisms upstream MCP-1 activation. The first involved insulin dependent phosphorylation of GATA2, a transcription factor crucial for adipogenesis and inflammatory program. In the second we showed that an increased expression of several inflammation markers, including MCP-1 in metabolic and vascular tissues might due to a deregulation of TNF-alpha Converting Enzyme (TACE). GATA-2 and TACE could be new targets in the treatment of obesity related inflammation and its complications.

Keywords: Obesity; Inflammation; Macrophage; Cytokine

1. Introduction

In recent years, obesity has emerged as a metabolic dysfunctional state characterized by chronic activation of proinflammatory pathways associated to macrophage infiltration within adipocytes, both playing a crucial role in the development of insulin resistance and cardiovascular diseases [1]. Thus, obesity has been hypotesized to be a proinflammatory state increasing the vulnerability of atherosclerotic plaques. Adipocytes, in addition to their storage functions, secreted many bioactive molecules, including cytokines, which are known to affect insulin sensitivity in other tissues [2]. Among these factors, many studies

* Corresponding author. Department of Internal Medicine, University of Rome Tor Vergata, Via Montpellier 1, 00133 Rome, Italy. Tel.: +39 0672596889; fax: +39 0672596890.
E-mail address: federicm@uniroma2.it (M. Federici).

doi:10.1016/j.ics.2007.04.002

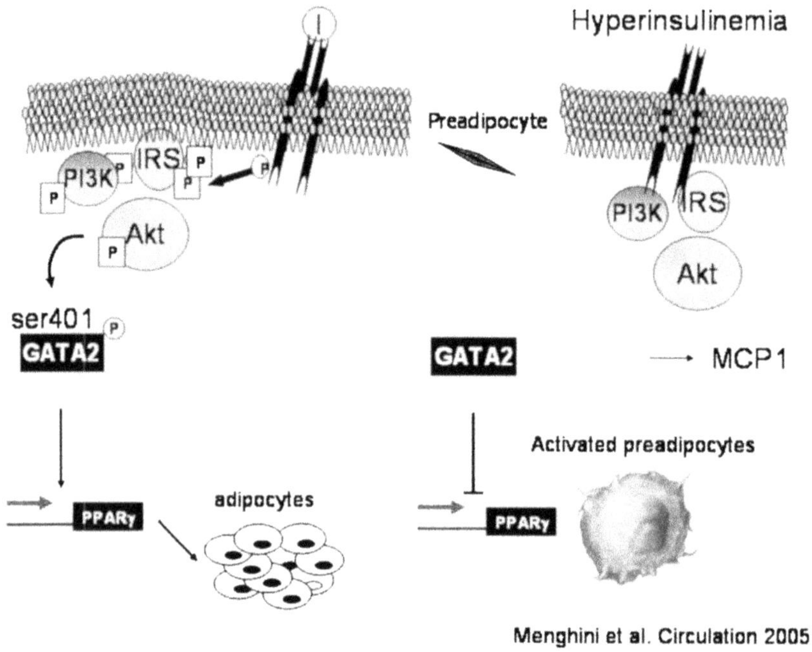

Fig. 1. Effect of GATA2 on preadipocytes.

have suggested that monocyte chemoattractant protein 1 (MCP-1) was a chemoattractant factor involved in the macrophages infiltration into adipose tissue, contributing to the development of obesity correlated complications. However, the signals that caused an increase in the expression of MCP-1 in adipocyte cells were still not clarified. On the other hand, it is established that MCP-1 plays a major role in regulating monocyte homing to atherosclerotic lesions. It is intriguing to hypothesize that similar mechanisms may modulate macrophage recruitment at multiple sites and contribute to the two most relevant complications of obesity, insulin resistance and cardiovascular diseases.

2. Macrophage recruitment

2.1. Macrophages and atherosclerosis

Atherogenesis is now recognized as a dynamic process that involves inflammation from the early stages of wall damage to the rupture of complicated (unstable) plaques [3]. Several studies have clearly shown that markers of inflammation are associated with atherosclerosis and ischemic heart disease [4,5], and that a range of mediators, such as cytokines and chemokines, are involved in the initiation of atherosclerotic lesions [6].

Macrophage cells played an essential role in the initiation and progression of atherosclerosis, and cells of monocytic origin were present in the developing foam cell lesion [7]. Experimental analyses with CD68 antibody staining have shown that macrophages infiltration occurred early in human atherosclerosis plaques. Migration of monocytes from the bloodstream to activated endothelial cells initially involved the recruitment of cells to the endothelium, followed by rolling along the vascular surface, adhesion and diapedesis between the tightly apposing endothelial cells, each process involving a large number of adhesion molecules. Then, monocytes migrated through the extracellular matrix of the tissues where they could differentiate into macrophages and reached the sites of inflammation. The macrophages recruitment was dependent on circulating monocyte levels and, although it is well established that blood monocytes, derived from bone marrow, are the source of arterial wall macrophages, the signals which initiate the recruitment and migration of monocytes to site of inflammation are not fully elucidated. Monocyte trafficking through the vessel wall was of current interest in the studies of pathogenesis of atherosclerosis and correlated diseases, such as diabetes and obesity.

2.2. Macrophages and obesity

In the classical view of the relationship between inflammation and insulin resistance adipocytes are believed to be the source of a large number of cytokines with a detrimental action on insulin sensitivity such as tumor necrosis factor-alpha (TNF-alpha), interleukin-6 (IL-6), monocyte chemoattractant protein-1 (MCP1), all proinflammatory molecules with a direct effect on cellular metabolism [8]. However, all these factors are generally released by activated macrophages in the context of an inflamed tissue. These overlapping properties of macrophages and adipocytes were explained considering the latter as a part of the innate immune system, To support this hypothesis is the observation that macrophages and adipocytes in the context of metabolic overload showed similar gene expression profiles and convergence of functions, such as lipid storage and cytokines secretion [8]. According to this hypothesis, the inflammatory burden of obesity and diabetes was therefore due to dysfunctional adipocytes, via the expression and release of cytokines like TNF-alpha and Interleukin-6.

In 2003 Weisberg et al. and Hu et al. [9,10] independently reported that both murine models and human samples of obesity are characterized by an increased number of macrophages within the adipose tissue, as assessed by the percentage of CD68+ cells, directly proportional to adipocyte size, supporting the hypothesis that adipocytes were not the source but the target of proinflammatory signals such as TNF-alpha, which derived from macrophages. During nutritional excess, unknown factors, produced within the adipose tissue caused monocyte recruitment and differentiation to activated macrophage. Furthermore, they observed that macrophages accumulation into the expanding adipose tissue was highly correlated with insulin resistance and metabolic syndrome. These two works challenged our vision of obesity-linked subclinical inflammation and adipose tissue macrophages were considered to be a major cause of obesity associated chronic inflammation. Macrophage-derived molecules might therefore act both locally on adipose tissue, and systemically on other organs, such as muscle, liver, beta cells [1]. However, which signals and pathways modulate the mechanism of macrophages recruitment to adipose tissue has not been clarified.

3. Role of chemokines in the macrophage recruitment: MCP-1

Emerging evidences suggested that chemotaxis played an important role in the recruitment of monocytes to inflammation site and several molecules with chemotactic activity have been described [11]. Among these, MCP-1 was one of the likely candidate, because of its expression in cells involved in atherogenesis and its increased activity in atherosclerotic lesions [12]. In vitro and in vivo experiments have shown that MCP-1 specifically attracted monocytes in a variety of pathological conditions, including atherosclerosis [13,14]. Recent studies in mouse models with increased susceptibility to atherosclerosis, have suggested a role of MCP-1 in the initiation of monocytes accumulation into atherosclerotic lesion. Deletion of MCP-1 gene in LDL receptor deficient mice, fed a high fat diet to induce fatty streaks, resulted in a dramatic reduction (83%) of lipid deposition and macrophages infiltration throughout the aortas, compared with wild type MCP-1 alleles mice [15]. Similarly, the absence of MCP-1 receptor (CCR2) in ApoE deficent mice, a model of severe atherosclerosis, decreased lesion formation in the aortic root, without affecting plasma lipid concentration [16]. In ApoB transgenic mice, MCP-1 deficiency resulted in the protection from foam cells formation [17], confirming a central role for the CCR2/MCP1 pathway in the recruitment of monocytes to early atherosclerotic lesions.

Interestingly, MCP-1 expression in adipose tissue has been found to positively correlate with obesity degree, both in human and animal models [18,19], and to increase earlier than other macrophage markers during the development of obesity [10] suggesting a potential role for MCP1 as a signal of monocytes recruitment into adipose tissue. Studies with MCP-1 homozygous knock down mice in diet induced obesity conditions have confirmed this hypothesis; in fact characterization of adipose tissue in this animal model led to the observation that body weight, adipocyte size and macrophage accumulation are reduced compared to wild type mice [20]. Furthermore, inhibition of MCP-1 functions protected from insulin resistance, glucose intolerance and hepatic steatosis associated with obesity, linking MCP-1 expression in obesity to correlate pathologies, by induction of an inflammatory response in adipose tissue.

3.1. CCR2/MCP-1 antagonists

Since treatments preventing macrophage infiltration into the adipose tissue might have a beneficial effect on the inflammatory response and metabolic pathologies, MCP-1 could represent a possible therapeutic target to treat obesity and its complications. Therefore, many studies have evaluated the effects of MCP-1 inactivation on progression of atherosclerotic lesions or in obesity models. To block the CCR2/MCP-1 signal pathway in vivo, an N-terminal deletion mutant of MCP-1 (7ND) has been created, which had a dominant negative function, forming an inactive heterodimer with endogenous mouse MCP-1 protein [21]. In ApoE deficient mice the 7ND gene expression was associated with a significant reduction in lesion progression and a decreased expression of MMP-9 and MMP-13, which are proteolytic enzymes involved in weakening the fibrous cap and promoting plaque rupture. These findings indicated that blockade of MCP-1 limited not only the plaque size, but also changed the lesion composition into a more stable phenotype, leading to reductions in thrombotic complications [22].

Acute inhibition of MCP-1 by 7ND expression in both db/db mice, a model of genetic obesity, and Diet-Induced Obesity (DIO) mice, significantly improved insulin resistance, glucose tolerance, and hepatic steatosis [20].

A comparable improvement in metabolic homeostasis was obtained by treating the same animal models with a selective small molecules antagonist of CCR2 [23]. Both MCP-1 or CCR2 inhibitions reduced the fraction of macrophage infiltration into adipose tissue of obese mice, correlating obesity induced inflammation with the perturbations associated to systemic glucose homeostasis.

4. CCR2/MCP-1 signaling regulation

In this scenario, a cross talk among adipocytes, macrophages and endothelial cells seemed to be crucial in the process of inflammation induced insulin resistance. Through MCP-1 secretion, adipocytes recruited macrophages to adipose tissue; in turn, the infiltrated macrophages directly influenced adipocyte biology, secreting many different chemokines or cytokines, which accounted for systemic insulin resistance [24]. It remained to be understood which signals regulated the increasing expression and secretion of MCP-1 in adipose tissue.

4.1. GATA-2 transcription factor

Data from our previous studies have shown that GATA-2, a transcription factor regulating hematopoietic differentiation, also expressed in a stromal vascular fraction of adipose tissue, was involved in the regulation of adipogenesis and macrophage recruitment, by controlling specific signals, including MCP-1 secretion in preadipocyte cells (Fig. 1) [25]. We found that insulin, the principal hormonal signal of adipogenesis, could inhibit GATA-2 activity, excluding it from the nucleus, through an Akt mediated phosphorylation on a specific site (Serine 401), thus enforcing the adipogenesis program. In fact, when a Serine 401 specific unphosphorylable mutant (GATA-2A) was expressed in preadipocytes, they lost their ability to differentiate both in vitro and in vivo, as shown by an oil red O staining assay of 3T3F442A cells in vitro and in vivo, using a fat pad formation model. Interestingly, GATA-2 phosphorylation on serine 401 also played a crucial role in the inflammatory pathway activation in preadipocytes. In vitro, as assessed by a cytokine protein array and mRNA analysis, GATA-2A preadipocytes if compared with preadipocytes transfected with a constitutively phosphorylated mutant (GATA-2D), expressed a significantly higher levels of macrophage-like cytokines, including MCP-1, but no increase in macrophage marker expression, indicating that preadipocytes blocked at a predifferentiation state may produce the most important chemokine for monocyte recruitment. In vivo, both MCP-1 and F4/80 mRNA were upregulated in fat pads derived from injection of GATA-2 and GATA-2A preadipocytes. Since GATA-2A does not increase the in vitro expression of F4/80 not expressed by preadipocytes, it could likely derive from macrophages migrated into fat pad in response to the increased MCP-1 expression. From this data, GATA-2 resulted to be an important gatekeeper of adipogenesis and early inflammatory signals in adipose tissue, regulating the expression of MCP-1 through an insulin dependent mechanism.

4.2. TIMP-3/TACE signaling

Regulation of TNF-alpha expression and release from metabolic tissues is believed to be a major determinant of insulin resistance [1]. TNF-alpha is also known to play a major

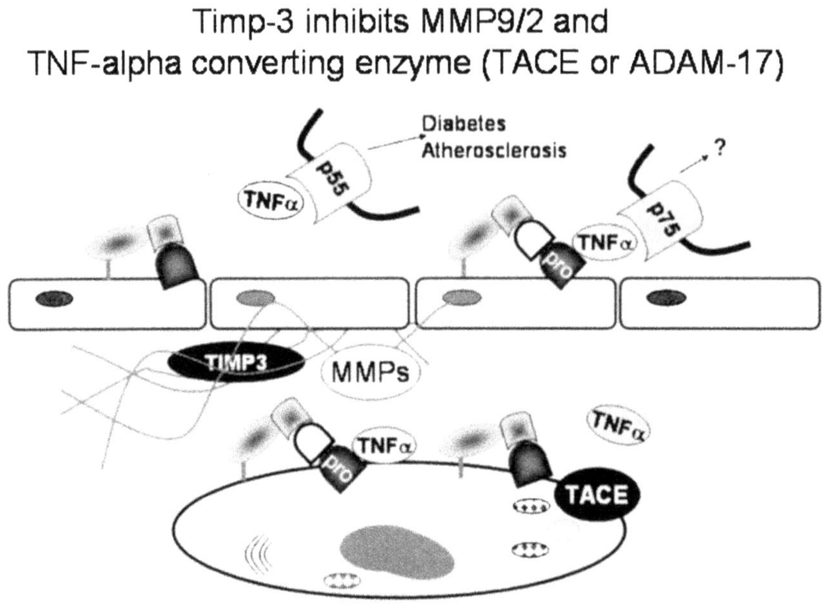

Fig. 2. Effect of TIMP3 on TACE and MMPs.

role in atherosclerosis progression [1]. TNF-alpha acts either in a paracrine manner as a soluble protein through its p55 receptor (TNFR1) or in an autocrine fashion, via interaction of the membrane TNF with TNFR2 (p75). The two receptors may result in different activities being the TNFR1/p55 the dominant one and the responsible for most of the negative effects of TNF-alpha on metabolic and vascular homeostasis. The ratio between the soluble and membrane TNF forms is regulated by the TNF-alpha Converting Enzyme, a metalloprotease belonging to the ADAM (A Disintegrin and A Metalloproteinase) family, also called ADAM17. ADAM17 is inhibited by another protein, known as Tissue Inhibitor of Metalloproteinase 3 (TIMP-3).

Interestingly, while searching for genetic modifiers of insulin resistance using the insulin receptor heterozygous mice (*Insr*$^{+/-}$), we found that Insr$^{+/-}$ mice that showed a diabetic phenotype, all exhibited an impaired expression of TIMP-3-gene [26]. TIMP-3, that is normally bound within the extracellular matrix [27], controlled different aspects of inflammatory complications inhibiting several matrix metalloproteinases (MMP) and ADAM's family members [28,29]. Loss of TIMP-3 impacted innate immune functions, by dysregulating cleavage of TNF-alpha and its receptor [30]. Our data showed that in skeletal muscle of *Insr*$^{+/-}$ diabetic mice, the reduction of TIMP-3 expression and activity correlated with an increased soluble form of TNF-alpha, due to an enhanced TACE activity, and increased expression of several inflammation markers, including MCP-1 [26]. In addition, we found that treatment of *Insr*$^{+/-}$ diabetic mice with MMP inhibitor-1 (TAPI-1), a synthetic inhibitor of TACE and MMPs, improved both glucose tolerance and inflammation. To investigate in details the role of TIMP-3 in modulating insulin action and vascular function, different mouse models were analyzed. *Insr*$^{+/-}$ *Timp3*$^{+/-}$ mice resulted to be more hyperinsulinemic and hyperglycaemic, in the fed state, compared with *Insr*$^{+/-}$, *Timp3*$^{+/-}$ or wild type mice, while TACE haploinsufficiency is associated with mildly increased insulin sensitivity, compared with wild type.

Treatment of *Insr*$^{+/-}$ mice with Timp3 deficiency and increased inflammation in the vascular tissues, with TAPI-1 led to a marked reduction of several markers of vascular damage such as Cox2 (oxidative stress), LOX-1 (oxLDL uptake), MCP-1 (monocyte recruitment) and VCAM-1 (monocyte adhesion to endothelium).

Interestingly, TIMP-3 was found to be downregulated in adipose tissue of genetic models of obesity [31].

Our laboratory is currently investigating whether TIMP-3, through TACE activation, is involved in the modulation of MCP-1 expression for the recruitment of macrophages in multiple metabolic and vascular tissues.

Our data provided an evidence that TACE activity, controlled by TIMP-3 signalling, might represent a regulator of glucose sensitivity and inflammatory pathways, via increased generation of soluble TNF-alpha and acting upstream to MCP-1 to drive macrophage homing, determining a mechanism for integration of metabolic and stress signals to different cell types, including adipocytes (Fig. 2).

References

[1] K.E. Wellen, G.S. Hotamisligil, Inflammation, stress, and diabetes, J. Clin. Invest. 115 (5) (2005) 1111–1119.

[2] K.E. Wellen, G.S. Hotamisligil, Obesity-induced inflammatory changes in adipose tissue, J. Clin. Invest. 112 (12) (2003) 1785–1788.

[3] R. Ross, Atherosclerosis — an inflammatory disease, N. Engl. J. Med. 340 (2) (1999) 115–126.

[4] P.M. Ridker, et al., C-reactive protein and other markers of inflammation in the prediction of cardiovascular disease in women, N. Engl. J. Med. 342 (12) (2000) 836–843.

[5] P.M. Ridker, et al., Plasma concentration of interleukin-6 and the risk of future myocardial infarction among apparently healthy man, Circulation 101 (15) (2000) 1767–1772.

[6] P. Libby, Current concepts of the pathogenesis of the acute coronary syndromes, Circulation 104 (3) (2001) 365–372.

[7] R. Ross, The pathogenesis of atherosclerosis: an update, N. Engl. J. Med. 314 (8) (1986) 488–500.

[8] M. Lehrke, M.A. Lazar, Inflamed about obesity, Nat. Med. 10 (2) (2004) 126–127.

[9] S.P. Weisberg, et al., Obesity is associated with macrophage accumulation in adipose tissue, J. Clin. Invest. 112 (12) (2002) 1796–1808.

[10] H. Xu, et al., Chronic inflammation in fat plays a crucial role in the development of obesity-related insulin resistance, J. Clin. Invest. 112 (12) (2002) 1821–1830.

[11] R.J. Aiello, et al., Monocyte chemoattractant protein 1 accelerates atherosclerosis in apolipoprotein E deficient mice, Arterioscler. Thromb. Vasc. Biol. 19 (6) (1999) 1518–1525.

[12] W. Peters, I.F. Charo, Involvement of chemokine receptor 2 and its ligand, monocyte chemoattractant protein 1, in the development of atherosclerosis: lessons from knockout mice, Curr. Opin. Lipidol. 12 (2) (2001) 175–180.

[13] M.E. Fuentes, et al., Controlled recruitment of monocytes/macrophages to specific organs through transgenic expression of MCP-1, J. Immunol. 155 (12) (1995) 5769–5776.

[14] M.D. Gunn, et al., Monocyte chemoattractant protein-1 is sufficient for the chemotaxis of monocytes and lymphocytes in transgenic mice but requires an additional stimulus for inflammatory activation, J. Immunol. 58 (1) (1997) 376–383.

[15] L. Gu, et al., Absence of monocyte chemoattractant protein-1 reduces atherosclerosis in low density lipoprotein receptor deficient mice, Mol. Cell 2 (2) (1998) 275–281.

[16] L. Boring, et al., Decreased lesion formation in CCR2−/−mice reveals a role for chemokines in the initiation of atherosclerosis, Nature 396 (6696) (1998) 894–897.

[17] J. Gosling, et al., MCP-1 deficiency reduces susceptibility to atherosclerosis in mice that overexpress human apolipoprotein B, J. Clin. Invest. 103 (6) (1999) 773–778.
[18] P. Sartipy, D.J. Loskutoff, Monocyte chemoattractant protein-1 in obesity and insulin resistance, Proc. Natl. Acad. Sci. U. S. A. 100 (12) (2003) 7265–7270.
[19] J.M. Bruun, et al., Monocyte chemoattractant protein-1 release is higher in visceral than subcutaneous human adipose tissue (AT): implication of macrophages resident in the AT, J. Clin. Endocrinol. Metab. 90 (4) (2005) 2282–2289.
[20] H. Kanda, et al., MCP-1 contributes to macrophage infiltration into adipose tissue, insulin resistance, and hepatic steatosis in obesità, J. Clin. Invest. 116 (6) (2006) 1494–1505.
[21] Y. Zhang, B.J. Rollins, A dominant negative inhibitor indicates that monocyte chemoattractant protein 1 functions as a dimer, Mol. Cell. Biol. 15 (9) (1995) 4851–4855.
[22] S. Inoue, K. Egashira, W. Ni, et al. Anti-monocyte chemoattractant protein-1 gene therapy limits progression and destabilization of established atherosclerosis in apolipoprotein E-knockout mice. Circulation;106 (21):2700–2706.
[23] S.P. Weisberg, et al., CCR2 mudulates inflammatory and metabolic effects of high fat feeding, J. Clin. Invest. 116 (1) (2006) 115–124.
[24] J.G. Neels, J.M. Olefsky, Inflamed fat: what starts the fire? J. Clin. Invest. 116 (1) (2006) 33–35.
[25] R. Menghini, et al., Phosphorylation of GATA2 by Akt increases adipose tissue differentiation and reduces adipose tissue related inflammation, Circulation 111 (15) (2002) 1946–1953.
[26] M. Federici, et al., TIMP3 deficiency in insulin receptor haploinsufficient mice promotes diabetes and vascular inflammation via increased TNF-α, J. Clin. Invest. 115 (12) (2005) 3494–3505.
[27] K.J. Leco, et al., Tissue inhibitor of metalloproteinases-3 (TIMP-3) is an extracellular matrix-associated protein with a distinctive pattern of expression in mouse cells and tissues, J. Biol. Chem. 269 (12) (1994) 9352–9360.
[28] G. Murphy, F. Willenbrock, Tissue inhibitors of matrix metalloendopeptidases, Methods Enzymol. 248 (1995) 496–510.
[29] A. Amour, et al., TNF-alpha converting enzyme (TACE) is inhibited by TIMP-3, FEBS Lett. 435 (1) (Sep 11 1998) 39–44.
[30] D.S. Smookler, et al., Tissue inhibitor of metalloproteinase 3 regulates TNF-dependent systemic inflammation, J. Immunol. 176 (2) (2006) 721–725.
[31] C. Chavey, et al., Matrix metalloproteinases are differently expressed in adipose tissue during obesity and modulate adipocyte differentiation, J. Biol. Chem. 278 (14) (2003) 11888–11896.

ELSEVIER

International Congress Series 1303 (2007) 31 – 34

www.ics-elsevier.com

Adipokines, systemic inflammation and inflamed adipose tissue in obesity and insulin resistance

Ulf Smith *, Christian X. Andersson, Birgit Gustafson, Ann Hammarstedt, Petter Isakson, Emelie Wallerstedt

The Lundberg Laboratory for Diabetes Research, Department of Molecular and Clinical Medicine/Diabetes, the Sahlgrenska Academy at Göteborg University, SE-413 45 Göteborg, Sweden

Abstract. Obesity and its complications are characterized by elevated circulating levels of inflammation markers like CRP, IL-6 and serum amyloid A.

Although several cells secrete these markers, the adipose tissue seems to play a pivotal role for the proinflammatory state. Obesity with enlarged adipose cells leads to a marked increase in the expression of pro-inflammatory cytokines in the adipose tissue while expression of the anti-inflammatory adipokine, adiponectin, is reduced. The mechanisms for this are currently unknown but a consequence is the recruitment of inflammatory cells into the adipose tissue which, thus, becomes inflamed. Animal experiments have shown that this is associated with a clear accentuation of degree of insulin resistance.

Invasion of inflammatory cells leads to the release of TNFa, which normally is not secreted by the adipose cells. The increased levels of cytokines in the adipose tissue have marked consequences for the normal differentiation of the preadipocytes. These cells become proinflammatory and the normal phenotype, i.e., lipid-accumulating and insulin-sensitive cells, is suppressed.

Although inflammation in the adipose tissue also leads to a reduced insulin sensitivity, recent data have shown that induction of insulin resistance by itself in the adipose tissue also is proinflammatory since insulin can exert an anti-inflammatory effect through its cross-talk with the IL-6 signaling cascade.

Keywords: Adipose tissue; Inflammation; Insulin resistance; Obesity; Type 2 diabetes; Cytokine

* Corresponding author. Tel.: +46 31 342 1104; fax: +46 31 829138.
E-mail address: ulf.smith@medic.gu.se (U. Smith).

doi:10.1016/j.ics.2007.03.015

1. Obesity, insulin resistance and inflammation

Many recent studies have shown that obesity, insulin resistance and Type 2 diabetes are proinflammatory states [1,2]. A number of different circulating markers of inflammation have been shown to be elevated as summarized in Table 1.

These markers are produced by different tissues and cells such as the endothelial and white blood cells, the liver and the adipose tissue. Since the degree of inflammation is related to future risks of developing Type 2 diabetes as well as cardiovascular disease [3,4], a key question is to understand how the proinflammatory state is induced. In addition, induction of inflammation is related to the development of insulin resistance [5].

2. What is the role of the adipose tissue?

Since obesity per se is a proinflammatory state, it is not unreasonable to attribute an important role to the adipose tissue. The best experimental demonstration of the importance of the adipose tissue for circulating IL-6 and serum amyloid A (SAA) levels, well-established markers of inflammation in man (Table 1), come from the engineered ATTAC mouse model [6]. This model is engineered to temporarily activate caspase-8 in the adipose tissue by administration of an activator/drug. This leads to the complete ablation of the adipose tissue in adult mice. Following withdrawal of the drug, the adipose tissue rapidly develops and this is probably a consequence of differentiating stem cells.

Using this model, it was clearly shown that the adipose tissue plays a key role for both the circulating IL-6 levels as well as the induction of SAA by endotoxins [6]. Also studies in man have shown that the adipose tissue is an important source of the circulating IL-6 levels [7] and that the adipose tissue interstitial fluid has considerably higher IL-6 levels than those seen in the circulation [8]. Taken together, currently available data clearly support a key role of the expanded adipose tissue for the proinflammatory state seen in obesity and its complications.

3. The adipose tissue is proinflammatory and inflamed in obesity

Obesity is associated with a gradual expansion of the adipose cells. These cells are remarkable in their ability to accommodate excess lipids for storage by varying the diameter

Table 1
Markers of subclinical inflammation are increased in type 2 diabetes and insulin resistance

- ❑ CRP
- ❑ Serum amyloid A
- ❑ α-1 Acid glycoprotein
- ❑ Haptoglobin
- ❑ Fibrinogen
- ❑ IL-6
- ❑ Soluble E-selection
- ❑ Soluble ICAM/VCAM-1
- ❑ PAI-1
- ❑ von Willebrand factor
- ❑ Leucocyte count

10- to 15-fold. Although functional for the storage of lipids, cell size expansion also leads to a reduction in the production of anti-inflammatory adipokines (like adiponectin) while proinflammatory cytokines (like IL-6) are markedly increased [9]. The reason for this is currently unknown but understanding this mechanism may provide new avenues for the development of anti-inflammatory agents.

It should be emphasized that the major source of proinflammatory adipokines is not the mature adipose cells but rather the stromal cells, in particular the preadipocytes and the invaded macrophages. Another consequence of the adipose cell expansion is to enhance the production of chemokines like IL-8 and MCP-1. This, in turn, leads to the infiltration of monocytes and macrophages into the adipose tissue [10].

Thus, obesity and adipose cell enlargement lead to the induction of proinflammatory cytokines and chemokines in the stromal cells, probably mainly by the committed but non-differentiated preadipocytes. This proinflammatory state is further enhanced by the infiltration of inflammatory cells from the blood into the adipose tissue.

4. Importance of the inflamed state of the adipose tissue in obesity

Animal experiments have shown that the induction of an inflamed state in the adipose tissue in obesity also coincides with the development of a pronounced insulin resistance.

The inflamed state leads to the release into the adipose tissue of cytokines that are not normally secreted by the adipose cells. A key cytokine that is released by macrophages, but not differentiated adipose cells, is TNFα. This key regulator of inflammation has pronounced effects on the preadipocytes by both inhibiting the normal differentiation and lipid accumulation by these cells as well as promoting a proinflammatory state [11]. Thus, the preadipocytes assume a different phenotype in the presence of TNFα which, in turn, is expected to augment both local and systemic inflammation [11].

5. Proinflammatory effect of insulin resistance in the adipose tissue

It is well established that induction of inflammation in the adipose tissue is associated with insulin resistance. However, recent work in our laboratory has shown that insulin resistance in the adipose cells also promotes the development of a proinflammatory state. Many studies have shown that obesity is associated with insulin resistance in the adipose tissue. Although there are probably several reasons for this, one important mechanism is likely to be the induction of a proinflammatory state in the adipose tissue as a consequence of the adipose cell enlargement. However, the insulin resistance cannot only antagonize the metabolic effects of insulin but also its recently documented anti-inflammatory effect. Recent work by Andersson et al. (unpublished) has shown that insulin antagonizes the proinflammatory effect of IL-6 through cross-talk with the signaling mechanisms for this cytokine. Thus, the inflamed adipose tissue associated with adipose cell enlargement in obesity can markedly promote both insulin resistance and inflammation through different local and systemic effects.

In conclusion, the adipose tissue plays a key role for the development of the proinflammatory and insulin-resistant state seen in obesity. Although we currently do not understand the molecular mechanisms involved, the expansion of the adipose cell size

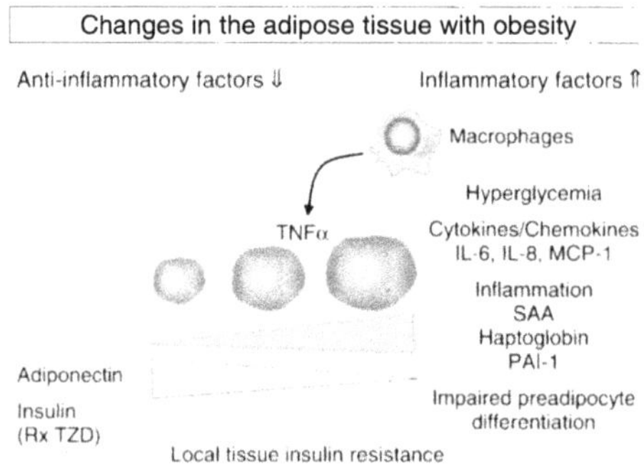

Fig. 1. Expansion of the adipose cells induces a proinflammatory state and recruitment of macrophages. This, in turn, leads to the release of TNFα which is a powerful antagonist of adipose cell differentiation while it promotes inflammation. Adiponectin, which is a marker of adipose cell differentiation, is reduced contributing to the insulin resistance both locally and systemically. The insulin resistance in the adipose tissue also promotes the proinflammatory state since insulin is anti-inflammatory in these cells. This effect is mediated by cross-talk with certain steps in the IL-6 signaling cascade.

seems to be a critical trigger of the subsequent series of events. Fig. 1 provides a schematic summary of the pro- and anti-inflammatory factors involved. The reduction of adiponectin secretion in obesity also contributes to the proinflammatory and insulin-resistant state.

References

[1] O.P. Kristiansen, T. Mandrup-Poulsen, Interleukin-6 and diabetes: the good, the bad, or the indifferent? Diabetes 54 (Suppl 2) (2005) S114–S124.

[2] P.A. Tataranni, E. Ortega, A burning question: does an adipokine-induced activation of the immune system mediate the effect of overnutrition on type 2 diabetes? Diabetes 54 (2005) 917–927.

[3] A.J. Hanley, et al., Metabolic and inflammation variable clusters and prediction of type 2 diabetes: factor analysis using directly measured insulin sensitivity, Diabetes 53 (2004) 1773–1781.

[4] A.D. Pradhan, et al., C-reactive protein, interleukin 6, and risk of developing type 2 diabetes mellitus, JAMA 286 (2001) 327–334.

[5] S.E. Shoelson, J. Lee, A.B. Goldfine, Inflammation and insulin resistance, J. Clin. Invest. 116 (2006) 1793–1801.

[6] U.B. Pajvani, et al., Fat apoptosis through targeted activation of caspase 8: a new mouse model of inducible and reversible lipoatrophy, Nat. Med. 11 (2005) 797–803.

[7] V. Mohamed-Ali, et al., Subcutaneous adipose tissue releases interleukin-6, but not tumor necrosis factor-alpha, in vivo, J. Clin. Endocrinol. Metab. 82 (1997) 4196–4200.

[8] V.R. Sopasakis, et al., High local concentrations and effects on differentiation implicate interleukin-6 as a paracrine regulator, Obes. Res. 12 (2004) 454–460.

[9] V. Rotter, I. Nagaev, U. Smith, Interleukin-6 (IL-6) induces insulin resistance in 3T3-L1 adipocytes and is, like IL-8 and tumor necrosis factor-alpha, overexpressed in human fat cells from insulin-resistant subjects, J. Biol. Chem. 278 (2003) 45777–45784.

[10] S.P. Weisberg, et al., Obesity is associated with macrophage accumulation in adipose tissue, J. Clin. Invest. 112 (2003) 1796–1808.

[11] B. Gustafson, U. Smith, Cytokines promote Wnt signaling and inflammation and impair the normal differentiation and lipid accumulation in 3T3-L1 preadipocytes, J. Biol. Chem. 281 (2006) 9507–9516.

International Congress Series 1303 (2007) 35–40
www.ics-elsevier.com

Oxidative stress, inflammation and atherosclerotic plaque development

Francesco Cipollone, Maria Luigia Fazia, Andrea Mezzetti *

Atherosclerosis, Hypertension and Dyslipidemia Unit, "G.d'Annunzio" University of Chieti-Pescara, Italy
Center for Aging Sciences, "G. d'Annunzio" University Foundation, Chieti-Pescara, Italy

Abstract. Although the pathophysiological mechanisms underlying atherosclerosis are not completely understood, it is widely recognized that both inflammation and oxidative stress play important roles in all of the phases of atherosclerosis evolution. The oxidative modification hypothesis of atherosclerosis supports the concept that oxidation of circulating low density lipoprotein (LDL) plays a key role in the early phases of atherogenesis. However, in addition to LDL oxidation, other oxidative events are worth noting in the setting of atherosclerosis, such as the generation of oxygen reactive species. These compounds are crucial mediators in the signaling pathways underlying vascular inflammation, from the initial phases of fatty streak formation to atherosclerotic plaque evolution toward instability and rupture. In this manuscript, we summarize the newest evidence linking oxidative signaling to inflammation and atherosclerosis evolution.

Keywords: Atherosclerosis; Inflammation; Oxidative stress

1. Introduction

Atherosclerosis is a complex disease in which the cellular and molecular mechanisms contributing to the disease process are not completely clear. However, increasing evidence in the last decades has clearly shown that atherosclerosis may be considered as a chronic inflammatory disease. Epidemiological studies have revealed a strong association between systemic inflammation and the future risk for symptomatic cardiovascular disease [1]. Moreover, the presence of inflammatory cells, i.e. macrophages and T lymphocytes, is already detectable in fatty streak, the first identifiable precursor of the atherosclerotic

* Corresponding author. Tel.: +39 0871 541339; fax: +39 0871 541337.
E-mail address: mezzetti@unich.it (A. Mezzetti).

0531-5131/
doi:10.1016/j.ics.2007.02.064

lesion, then increases with plaque progression, and finally characterizes the sites of ruptured plaques. In fact, unstable plaques typically contain a greater inflammatory area with respect to stable plaques, and this strongly supports the crucial role of inflammation in plaque instability [2].

Recently, it has been proposed that inflammation may be considered the mechanistical link between the well-established risk factors for the development of atherosclerosis and atherogenesis. In particular, emerging data have shown that a common pathologic mechanism shared by hyperlipidemia, hypertension, smoking, diabetes, could lead to generation of oxidative milieu that modulate, in turn, the inflammatory state of vascular wall genes [3]. In this paper, we summarize the pathophysiology of atherosclerosis, focusing on the role of pathways linking oxidative stress and inflammation in this setting.

2. Endothelial dysfunction and atherogenesis

The endothelium is a continuous layer of cells that separates blood from the vessel wall; it manifests a variety of phenotypes that vary between vascular beds. An active, dynamic tissue, the endothelium controls many important functions, including maintenance of blood circulation and fluidity as well as regulation of vascular tone, coagulation, and inflammatory responses [4]. The arterial endothelium responds to flow and shear forces via a pathway that leads to phosphorylation of endothelial nitric oxide synthase (eNOS), which produces nitric oxide ($NO^{\cdot}$) and thus leads to vasodilation. This response allows conduit arteries to accommodate increases in flow and control changes in shear. In addition, the endothelium limits local thrombosis by producing tissue plasminogen activator, maintaining a negatively charged surface, and secreting heparans and thrombomodulin [5].

Endothelial cells (EC) dysfunction occurs when the cell loses its ability to maintain the normal homeostatic balance, ultimately leading to impairment in vasorelaxation and increased adhesiveness of the endothelium lining for circulating inflammatory cells [4]. Indeed, when the arterial endothelium encounters certain bacterial products or risk factors as diverse as dyslipidemia, vasoconstrictor hormones inculpated in hypertension, the products of glycoxidation associated with hyperglycemia, or proinflammatory cytokines derived from excess adipose tissue, these cells augment the expression of adhesion molecules that promote the sticking of blood leukocytes to the inner surface of the arterial wall [6]. The most important adhesion molecules are intercellular adhesion molecule-1 (ICAM-1) and vascular adhesion molecule-1 (VCAM-1) and selectins. ICAM-1 and VCAM-1 regulate attachment and transendothelial migration of leukocytes. Both macrophages and endothelial cells produce ICAM-1 in response to inflammatory cytokines such as IL-1, TNF-α, and interferon-γ, whereas VCAM-1 expression is mainly restricted to endothelial cells. Cytokine-stimulated endothelial cells also produce monocyte chemotactic protein-1 (MCP-1), monocyte colony-stimulating factor, and IL-6, which further amplifies the inflammatory cascade [7]. The selectins are adhesion molecules that mediate the initial rolling of inflammatory cells along endothelial cells and platelets.

Once resident in the arterial intima, the blood leukocytes–mainly mononuclear phagocytes and T lymphocytes–communicate with endothelial and smooth muscle cells

(SMCs), the endogenous cells of the arterial wall. As a major consequence of the inflammatory ferment underway in the early atheroma, SMCs migrate from the tunica media into the intima. These cells proliferate and elaborate a rich and complex extracellular matrix. In concert with endothelial cells and monocytes, they secrete matrix metalloproteinases (MMPs) in response to various oxidative, hemodynamic, inflammatory, and autoimmune signals. MMPs, in balance with their endogenous tissue inhibitors, modulate numerous functions of vascular cells, including activation, proliferation, migration, and cell death, as well as new vessel formation, geometric remodeling, healing, or destruction of extracellular matrix of arteries and the myocardium [8].

As the atheromatous plaque matures, it develops a fibrous cap and lipid core. The vulnerable plaque is characterized by a thin fibrous cap and large lipid pool. Interstitial collagen, produced by smooth muscle cells, confers tensile strength and stability to the fibrous cap. Platelet-derived growth factor, released by platelets during thrombosis, and transforming growth factor-β, increases the rate of collagen production. Conversely, macrophages, in response to stimulation by T cells, can produce MMPs, which actively break down the collagen and other extracellular matrix proteins in the fibrous cap. T cells may also produce interferon-γ, which signals to smooth muscle cells to decrease collagen synthesis. Thus a dynamic balance is maintained between collagen synthesis and breakdown. If the equilibrium is tipped to a proinflammatory state, fibrous cap thinning and eventual rupture may result [9].

3. A common mechanism linking cardiovascular risk factors: oxidative stress?

Hyperlipidemia, diabetes, hypertension, and smoking are well-established risk factors for the development of atherosclerosis. However, the molecular and cellular mechanisms linking these diverse risk factors to a common pathologic mechanism are unclear. A current hypothesis suggests that modulation of the expression of a selective set of vascular inflammatory genes by intracellular oxidative signals may provide a molecular mechanism linking these seemingly diverse risk factors with the early pathogenesis of atherosclerosis [3,10]. As such, various proinflammatory or prooxidant stimuli associated with these risk factors may directly stimulate or sensitize vascular cells to generate ROS. These ROS and/or their modified target biomolecules (i.e., oxidized LDL) then serve as true second-messenger coupling molecules to transmit these extracellular signals to elevated expression of atherogenic gene products such as adhesion molecules and other vascular inflammatory gene products. The induced expression of these gene products thus promotes the infiltration of monocytes into the vessel wall and the release of additional proinflammatory signals. Accordingly, this positive feedback loop would serve to potentiate the local inflammatory response and endothelial cell dysfunction. However, mammalian cells are protected from ROS by antioxidant defense mechanisms such as the enzymes catalase, superoxide dismutase (SOD), and glutathione peroxidase (GPx). When the normal redox homeostasis of the cell is upset and the rate of formation of ROS exceeds the capacity of the antioxidant defense system, a condition of oxidative stress occurs. Despite the experimental evidence implicating redox processes and oxidative stress in the pathogenesis of atherosclerosis, little is known about the relative role of each of the potential sources for ROS production in the vasculature.

Because of the apparent importance of ROS in vascular disease, there has been substantial interest in the enzymatic sources that contribute to production of free radicals in vascular tissues. Several enzyme systems seem to be important in this process, including xanthine oxidase, the nicotinamide adenine dinucleotide phosphate (NADPH) oxidases, mitochondrial sources, and nitric oxide synthase (NOS) [11]. In brief, these enzymes use various substrates as sources of electrons that subsequently reduce molecular oxygen to form a variety of ROS. A 1-electron reduction of oxygen leads to production of superoxide, and a 2-electron oxidation of oxygen leads to formation of hydrogen peroxide. Dismutation of superoxide, by superoxide dismutase can also lead to formation of hydrogen peroxide. A myriad of other ROS can be derived from superoxide and hydrogen peroxide, including lipid radicals, carbon-centered radicals, thiyl radicals, the hydroxyl radical, and hypochlorous acid. Some of these are formed by actions of peroxidases and by peroxidase actions of the copper/zinc superoxide dismutases.

4. Oxidative stress and vascular function

It is now recognized that the production of ROS and the resultant oxidative stress play a key role in mediating the pathologic manifestations of EC dysfunction associated with atherosclerosis. Indeed, endothelial dysfunction is associated to an impairment of endothelium-dependent vasorelaxation caused by a loss of nitric oxide ($NO^{\cdot}$) bioactivity in the vessel wall. A decline in $NO^{\cdot}$ bioavailability may be caused by decreased expression of the endothelial cell $NO^{\cdot}$ synthase (eNOS), a lack of substrate or cofactors for eNOS, alterations of cellular signaling such that eNOS is not appropriately activated, and, finally, accelerated $NO^{\cdot}$ degradation by ROS [12]. Under physiological conditions, endogenous antioxidant defenses minimize this interaction and maintain what seems to be a tenuous balance between $O_2^{-\cdot}$ and $NO^{\cdot}$.

This tenuous balance seems to be altered in a variety of common disease states. One of the first examples of this came from studies of hypercholesterolemic rabbits. These animals have severely impaired endothelium-dependent vascular relaxation, suggesting a lack of $NO^{\cdot}$. Paradoxically, the production of total nitrogen oxides ($NO^{\cdot}$ and oxidation products of $NO^{\cdot}$) was increased by as much as 3-fold in these vessels. Furthermore, nitrogen oxide production increased appropriately on stimulation with either acetylcholine or the calcium ionophore A23187, suggesting that signaling pathways leading to eNOS activation were intact in these vessels [13]. These findings led to the speculation that hypercholesterolemia could result in oxidation of $NO^{\cdot}$ to vaso-inactive nitrogen oxides (such as nitrite and nitrate). Subsequently, it was shown that treatment of cholesterol-fed rabbits with polyethylene–glycolated-SOD could markedly enhance endothelium-dependent vascular relaxation but have no effect in normocholesterolemic animals [14]. This observation strongly supported the concept that in hypercholesterolemia, nitric oxide bioavailability is reduced by $O_2^{-\cdot}$.

Subsequently, altered endothelium-dependent vascular relaxation has been associated with enhanced degradation of $NO^{\cdot}$ by ROS in animal models of many different diseases. These include hypertension, diabetes, cigarette smoking, and heart failure. These studies have been extended to humans. Antioxidant vitamins have been shown to enhance endothelium-dependent vasodilation in both the coronary and forearm circulations in subjects with many of the same diseases examined in animal models [15].

Among ROS that can react with NO˙, superoxide is probably one of the most important. However, lipid radicals (LO˙ and LOO˙) also can react with NO˙ to form, respectively, LONO and LOONO. It is of interest that oxidized LDL, but not native LDL, added to isolated vessels inhibits endothelium-dependent vascular relaxation [16]. The oxidation of LDL leads to production of linoleic hydroperoxy and alkoxy radicals that could participate in such reactions with NO˙.

ROS also increase monocyte adhesion, cause EC apoptosis, and play a role in angiogenesis. The endothelium normally presents an inert inflammatory surface. However, many proinflammatory stimuli induce the expression of adhesion molecules on ECs, leading to monocyte adhesion and ultimately atherosclerotic lesion formation. Expression of several adhesion molecules, including VCAM-1 and ICAM-1, is ROS-dependent. Interleukin-1β and TNF-α-induced VCAM-1 gene expression is suppressed by the antioxidants pyrrolidine dithiocarbamate (PDTC) and NAC [17]. Furthermore, NO˙, which, because of its ability to scavenge radicals, can act as an antioxidant and reduces VCAM-1 expression stimulated by TNF-α, possibly by inhibiting the formation of peroxy-fatty acids. Induction of VCAM-1 and ICAM-1 expression by oscillatory shear stress is also inhibited by NAC [18]. Taken together, these observations suggest that ROS promote adhesion of inflammatory cells.

Endothelial injury or exposure to $O_2^{\bullet -}$ and H_2O_2 induces apoptosis of ECs, which leads to EC loss and results in atherogenesis and a procoagulative state [19]. Importantly, EC apoptosis stimulated by oxidized LDL, Ang II, high glucose, and TNF-α is inhibited by SOD, catalase, NAC, and antioxidant vitamins. These data strongly suggest that ROS regulate apoptotic mechanisms induced by a variety of stimuli. Another type of programmed cell death, anoikis, results from detachment of ECs from extracellular matrix. This process is also associated with increased intracellular ROS, probably from mitochondria, and is inhibited by NAC and diphenylene iodonium (DPI), a inhibitor of flavin-containing enzymes such as NAD(P)H oxidases.

ROS production is also implicated in angiogenesis, a process important not only for physiological processes such as embryonic development and wound repair but also for pathological processes such as cancer, diabetic retinopathy, and atherosclerosis. EC migration, proliferation, and tube formation are essential events in the process of angiogenesis. ROS may be directly involved in all these mechanisms, as H_2O_2 has been shown to induce proliferation and migration of ECs and to mediate lymphocyte-activated tubulogenesis [20]. ROS also act as mediators of angiogenic growth factors, such as vascular endothelial growth factor (VEGF). It has been reported that NAD(P)H oxidases regulate not only the induction of VEGF expression but also VEGF-induced angiogenesis [21].

ROS generation is also involved in modulation of many functions of VSMCs. Perhaps the most well-studied of these processes is cell growth, but ROS are also involved in migration as well as expression of inflammatory mediators and matrix components. In addition, ROS have been implicated in VSMC contraction. Synthetic VSMCs, whose phenotype has been altered to support growth, are found in cardiovascular diseases such as hypertension, atherosclerosis, and restenosis after balloon angioplasty. ROS production is intimately involved in many of the processes leading to both hypertrophic and proliferative VSMC growth.

5. Conclusions

It has been recognized that atherosclerosis is an inflammatory disease linked to an abnormality in oxidation-mediated signals in the vascular system. Understanding the molecular basis of the processes implicated in redox-sensitive vascular gene expression could contribute to elucidate the complex pathogenesis of atherosclerosis and to identify novel pharmacological approaches.

References

[1] P. Libby, P.M. Ridker, A. Maseri, Inflammation and atherosclerosis, Circulation 105 (9) (2002) 1135–1143.
[2] F. Cipollone, et al., Overexpression of functionally coupled cyclooxygenase-2 and prostaglandin E synthase in symptomatic atherosclerotic plaques as a basis of prostaglandin E(2)-dependent plaque instability, Circulation 104 (8) (2001) 921–927.
[3] C. Kunsch, R.M. Medford, Oxidative stress as a regulator of gene expression in the vasculature, Circ. Res. 85 (8) (1999) 753–766.
[4] A.M. Gonzalez, A.P. Selwyn, Endothelial function, inflammation, and prognosis in cardiovascular disease, Am. J. Med. 115 (8A) (2003) 99S–106S.
[5] D. Behrendt, P. Ganz, Endothelial function: from vascular biology to clinical applications, Am. J. Cardiol. 90 (2002) 40L–48L (suppl).
[6] P. Libby, Vascular biology of atherosclerosis: overview and state of the art, Am. J. Cardiol. 91 (3A) (2003) 3A–6A.
[7] J.G. Blake, P.M. Ridker, Novel clinical markers of vascular wall inflammation, Circ. Res. 89 (9) (2001) 763–771.
[8] H. Nagase, R. Visse, G. Murphy, Structure and function of matrix metalloproteinases and TIMPs, Cardiovasc. Res. 69 (3) (2006) 562–573.
[9] F. Cipollone, M. Fazia, A. Mezzetti, Novel determinants of plaque instability, J. Thromb. Haemost. 3 (9) (2005) 1962–1975.
[10] R.W. Alexander, Theodore Cooper Memorial Lecture. Hypertension and the pathogenesis of atherosclerosis: oxidative stress and the mediation of arterial inflammatory response: a new perspective, Hypertension 25 (2) (1995) 155–161.
[11] D. Harrison, et al., Role of oxidative stress in atherosclerosis, Am. J. Cardiol. 91 (3A) (2003) 7A–11A.
[12] D.G. Harrison, Endothelial function and oxidant stress, Clin. Cardiol. 20 (11 Suppl 2) (1997) II-11-7.
[13] R.L. Minor, et al., Diet-induced atherosclerosis increases the release of nitrogen oxides from rabbit aorta, J. Clin. Invest. 86 (6) (1990) 2109–2116.
[14] A. Mugge, et al., Chronic treatment with polyethylene-glycolated superoxide dismutase partially restores endothelium-dependent vascular relaxations in cholesterol-fed rabbits, Circ. Res. 69 (5) (1991) 1293–1300.
[15] U. Solzbach, et al., Vitamin C improves endothelial dysfunction of epicardial coronary arteries in hypertensive patients, Circulation 96 (5) (1997) 1513–1519.
[16] F.C. Tanner, et al., Oxidized low density lipoproteins inhibit relaxations of porcine coronary arteries: role of scavenger receptor and endothelium-derived nitric oxide, Circulation 83 (6) (1991) 2012–2020.
[17] N. Marui, et al., Vascular cell adhesion molecule-1 (VCAM-1) gene transcription and expression are regulated through an antioxidant-sensitive mechanism in human vascular endothelial cells, J. Clin. Invest. 92 (4) (1993) 1866–1874.
[18] D.C. Chappell, et al., Oscillatory shear stress stimulates adhesion molecule expression in cultured human endothelium, Circ. Res. 82 (5) (1998) 532–539.
[19] S. Dimmeler, A.M. Zeiher, Reactive oxygen species and vascular cell apoptosis in response to angiotensin II and pro-atherosclerotic factors, Regul. Pept. 90 (1–3) (2000) 19–25.
[20] N. Maulik, D.K. Das, Redox signaling in vascular angiogenesis, Free Radic. Biol. Med. 33 (8) (2002) 1047–1060.
[21] M. Ushio-Fukai, et al., Novel role of gp91(phox)-containing NAD(P)H oxidase in vascular endothelial growth factor-induced signaling and angiogenesis, Circ. Res. 91 (12) (2002) 1160–1167.

International Congress Series 1303 (2007) 41 – 47
ELSEVIER
www.ics-elsevier.com

Insulin signaling in hypertension

Bruno Trimarco *, Salvatore Crispo, Carmine Morisco

Dipartimento di Medicina Clinica Scienze Cardiovascolari ed Immunologiche Università FEDERICO II, Via S. Pansini n. 5,80131 Napoli, Italy

Abstract. Insulin resistance has been described in several diseases that increase cardiovascular risk and mortality, such as diabetes mellitus, obesity, essential hypertension, metabolic syndrome, and heart failure. In last years it has been clarified the role of insulin resistance in the pathogenesis of hypertension and target organ damage. Dysregulation of sympathetic nervous and renin–angiotensin systems resulting in enhanced stimulation of both adrenergic (ARs) and angiotensin II receptors (AT) are typical features of hypertension. Overactivity of the renin–angiotensin system observed in hypertension is likely to impair insulin signaling and contribute to insulin resistance. Actually, Ang II acting through the AT1 receptor inhibits the actions of insulin in vascular tissue, in part, by interfering with insulin signaling through PI3K and downstream Akt signaling pathways via generation of reactive oxygen species (ROS) by NADPH oxidase. On the contrary, stimulation of βARs is able to induce insulin resistance through the activation of different serine/threonine kinases that blunt the insulin signal by phosphorylating IR or IRS-1. Hypertension is also associated with an endothelial chronic inflammatory response characterized by altered cytokine production and activation of inflammatory signaling pathways, this activation results in an impairment of insulin signaling. Understanding the molecular mechanisms which can interfere with the impairment insulin signalling may be useful to improve blood pressure control as well as cardiac and cerebral protection in hypertension.

Keywords: Glucose uptake; Protein kinase B; Adrenergic receptors; Angiotensin II; Oxidative stress

1. Insulin resistance and cardiovascular risk

Insulin resistance is defined as a less than expected biological response to a given concentration of the hormone and plays a pivotal role in the pathogenesis of type II diabetes

* Corresponding author.
E-mail address: trimarco@unina.it (B. Trimarco).

0531-5131/
doi:10.1016/j.ics.2007.04.005

mellitus [1]. Moreover, insulin resistance has been described in several diseases that increase cardiovascular risk and mortality, such as obesity [2], hypertension [3], metabolic syndrome [4], and heart failure [5,6]. Over the last decade, the link between insulin resistance and cardiovascular risk was exclusively attributed to the development of atherosclerosis. In fact, insulin resistance is thought to promote atherosclerosis, in part through associated metabolic abnormalities, hyperglycemia, hyperinsulinemia, and dyslipidemia, which stimulate smooth muscle cell hypertrophy and hyperplasia, and increase synthesis of extracellular matrix proteins. However, in the last years, it became evident that insulin resistance is not merely a problem of impaired glucose homeostasis, but a complex and multifaceted syndrome that can affect different organs or tissues with different pathophysiologycal consequences. For instance, in the context of the vascular system, it has been demonstrated that insulin stimulation induces vasodilation through nitric oxide (NO) production [7] and the state of "insulin resistance" impairs NO synthesis and vasodilation.

2. Molecular mechanisms of insulin resistance

In the last years, the pathophysiological mechanisms that during insulin resistance contribute to the development of cardiovascular diseases have become clearer. Abnormalities of insulin signaling account for insulin resistance. Insulin mediates its action on target organs through phosphorylation of a transmembrane-spanning tyrosine kinase receptor, the insulin receptor (IR). Binding of insulin to the α subunit of its receptor activates the tyrosine kinase activity of the β subunit of the receptor [8] leading to autophosphorylation, as well as, tyrosine phosphorylation of several IR substrates (IRS) including IRS1 and IRS2. These, in turn, interact with phosphatidylinositol 3-kinase (PI 3-kinase). Activation of PI 3-kinase stimulates the main downstream effector Akt (also called as protein kinase B) a serine/theronine kinase, which stimulates the glucose uptake in vascular, skeletal muscle and adipose tissue [9,10], and induce vasorelaxation by mechanisms that include the production of nitric oxide (NO). Several mechanisms have been described as responsible for the inhibition of insulin-stimulated tyrosine phosphorylation of IR and the IRS proteins, including proteasome-mediated degradation [11], phosphatase-mediated dephosphorylation [12], and kinase-mediated serine/treonine phoshporylation [13]. In particular, phosphorylation of IRS-1 on serine Ser612 causes dissociation of the p85 subunit of PI3-K, inhibiting further signalling. In addition, phosphorylation of IRS-1 on Ser307 results in its dissociation from the insulin receptor and triggers proteasome-dependent degradation, also impairing insulin signaling.

3. Insulin resistance directly affects blood pressure control

In last years it has been clarified the role of insulin resistance in the pathogenesis of hypertension and target organ damage. For instance, in healthy subjects insulin evokes a net reflex in sympathetic outflow, and at the same time it is able to blunt the vasoconstrictive effect resulting from this sympathetic activation. On the contrary, in hypertensive patients insulin evokes a sympathetic activation that is three times greater than that evoked in normal subject, and, at the same time, its vasorelaxant action is impaired [14]. This mechanism is involved in dysregulation of peripheral vascular resistance, which contributes to increase in blood pressure levels. The key role of insulin resistance in the pathogenesis of hypertension has been further supported by the evidence that in aortic rings of spontaneously hypertensive rats (SHR) the resistance to the vascular action of insulin is already present at the age of 5 weeks, before the onset of arterial hypertension [15], suggesting that in SHR the vascular resistance to insulin action is specific and not related to the compensatory hyperinsulinemia or hyperglycemia.

The mechanistic role of abnormalities of IR or IRS-1 signaling in the pathogenesis of insulin resistance and hypertension is supported by several studies performed in genetically engineered mice. In particular, transgenic mice with targeted disruption of the IRS-1 gene, exhibited higher blood pressure and plasma triglyceride levels compared to wild-type mice. They also showed an impairment of endothelium-dependent vascular relaxation [16]. On the other hand, mice heterozygous for knockout of the IR showed fasting blood glucose, insulin, free fatty acid, and triglyceride levels similar to those of wild-type mice. Interestingly, these mice had increased systolic blood pressure and blunted insulin-stimulated aortic endothelial nitric oxide synthase (NOS) phosphorylation [17]. The results of these studies allow to speculate that the abnormalities of IR or IRS signaling contribute to the development of hypertension risk independently form glucose homeostasis and plasma insulin levels. Accordingly, insulin resistance by itself is involved the pathogenesis of hypertension.

4. Insulin resistance and hypertension

It has been demonstrated that there is impaired insulin signaling in essential hypertension. In recent years, it has become evident that phenomenon of insulin resistance is tissue-specific and depend upon the type of stress, therefore, insulin receptor defects in specific tissues do not necessarily confer systemic insulin resistance. For instance, insulin resistance has be found in rodents with genetic hypertension such as Zucker obese and Goto-Kakizaki rats [18,19]. On the contrary, we have found that SHR have a normal insulin sensitivity in skeletal muscle compared the normotensive rat strain [20], but impaired cardiac insulin sensitivity. At molecular level, we found that, in the heart, insulin is able to induce tyrosine phosphorylation of its receptor to a similar extent in SHR and in normotensive control rats WKY. In the contrast, in SHR IRS-1 tyrosine phosphorylation was found markedly increased in basal conditions and paradoxically decreased after insulin exposure. This was associated with decreased association between IRS-1 and p85 regulatory subunit of PI 3-kinase, and PI3K activity in response to insulin stimulation.

Dysregulation of sympathetic nervous [21] and renin–angiotensin systems resulting in enhanced stimulation of both adrenergic (ARs) and angiotensin II receptors (AT) are typical features of hypertension. In vivo and in vitro studies have shown that angiotensin II (Ang II) stimulation also induces insulin resistance. Interventional studies have documented that angiotensin converting enzyme (ACE) inhibitors [22] and angiotensin type 1 receptor blockers (ARBr)[23] reduce the incidence of diabetes mellitus. Therefore, overactivity of the renin–angiotensin system observed in hypertension is likely to impair insulin signaling and contribute to insulin resistance. More recently, it has been reported that an ACE-inhibitor based long term treatment does not reduce the occurrence of diabetes mellitus in subjects impaired glucose tolerance [24]. This observation suggests that the pathophysiological mechanisms underlying the development of insulin resistance in hypertensive patients are different from those that account for impaired insulin sensitivity in diabetics.

Actually, Ang II acting through the AT1 receptor inhibits the actions of insulin in vascular tissue, in part, by interfering with insulin signaling through PI3K and downstream Akt signaling pathways via generation of reactive oxygen species (ROS) by NADPH oxidase [25]. ROS are important intracellular second messengers. Recent studies have demonstrated that the generation of ROS is implicated in the Ang II-induced insulin resistance. In this regard it has been demonstrated that in vascular smooth muscle cells isolated from rat thoracic aorta Ang II profoundly decreases IRS-1 protein levels via ROS-mediated phosphorylation of IRS-1 on Ser307 and subsequent proteasome-dependent degradation [26]. The key role of ROS in the pathogenesis of Ang II-induced insulin resistance has been also confirmed by in vivo studies. In particular, in rats chronic infusion of Ang II induced hypertension and reduced insulin-induced glucose uptake during hyperinsulinemic–euglycemic clamp, and increased plasma cholesterylester hydroperoxide levels, indicating an increased oxidative stress. Treatment with tempol, a superoxide dismutase mimetic, normalized plasma cholesterylester hydroperoxide levels in AII-infused rats. In addition, tempol normalized insulin resistance in AII-infused rats, as well as enhanced insulin-induced PI 3-kinase activation, suggesting that Ang II-induced insulin resistance can be restored by removing the oxidative stress [27]. On the other hand, in the endothelial cells, Ang II induces insulin resistance through the phosphorylation of IRS-1 at Ser312 and Ser616 via JNK- and ERK1/2-dependent mechanisms, respectively. This impairs the interaction of IRS-1 with the p85 regulatory subunit of PI 3-kinase and compromises the insulin vasodilatory signaling pathway involving PI 3-kinase/Akt/eNOS [28]. Altogether, these observations provide clear insight into the pathogetic mechanisms of Ang II-induced insulin resistance in the development of hypertension.

It has been documented that increased sympathetic tone resulting in an abnormal stimulation of βARs is able to induce insulin resistance through the activation of different serine/threonine kinases that blunt the insulin signal by phosphorylating IR or IRS-1. In recent years it has become evident that the molecular mechanisms that account for β ARs-induced insulin resistance are tissue-specific and depend upon the receptor subtype expressed. For instance, adipocytes and cardiac myocytes are both target organs of insulin, and mainly express β3 and β1 ARs, respectively. β AR stimulation results in an impairment of insulin signaling and insulin-induced glucose uptake, which profoundly differs between the two cell types regarding the kinetic and molecular mechanisms involved. In particular, β AR stimulation in adipocytes impairs insulin signaling within few minutes, whereas, in cardiac myocytes stimulation of β AR has a biphasic effect on insulin-stimulated glucose uptake, with an initial additive, followed by an inhibitory action. β3 AR stimulation impairs insulin signaling through a protein kinase A (PKA) - and protein kinase C (PKC)-dependent mechanisms; interestingly β3 AR stimulation does not phosphorylate/activate Akt [29]. On the contrary, in cardiac myocytes Akt plays a key role in the cross-talk between β1 AR and IR. Actually, upon the phosphorylation site, Akt can have a favourable or detrimental effect on insulin signaling and insulin-induced glucose uptake. In particular, short-term β AR stimulation induces Akt phosphorylation in threonine that results in an increase in glucose uptake, whereas long-term stimulation induces Akt phosphorylation in serine and impairs insulin evoked-glucose uptake and insulin-induced tyrosine autophosporylation of IR [30]. In addition, it has been recently demonstrated in cardiac myocytes, that chronic Akt activation is sufficient to impair insulin signal by inducing IRS-1 phosphorylation and proteasome-dependent degradation [31].

In the last decade, it has been clearly demonstrated that oxidative stress and endothelial cell inflammation directly trigger the development of a proinflammatory and proatherosclerotic state, leading to atherothrombosis. At this regard, it has been demonstrated that insulin, on one hand, suppresses the activity of different molecular pathways involved in development of atherosclerosis, and on the other hand, increases the expression and the activities of pathways with antiatherosclerotic action. Actually, insulin interferers with NF-κB binding activity, and, at the same time, increases IκB expression in mononuclear cells (MNCs). Furthermore, insulin has been shown to suppress plasma concentrations of intercellular adhesion molecule-1 and monocyte chemotactic protein-1 [32]. In addition, insulin suppresses activating protein-1 (AP-1) and Egr-1, two pro-inflammatory transcription factors and their respective genes, matrix metalloproteinase-9, tissue factor (TF), and PAI-1 [33]. Thus, insulin has a comprehensive antiinflammatory effect. An impairment of the action of insulin due to insulin resistance would thus result in the activation of these proinflammatory factors and increase the risk for atherothrombosis. Hypertension is associated with an endothelial chronic inflammatory response characterized by altered cytokine production and activation of inflammatory signaling pathways. Recent reports have linked this inflammatory response to the development of insulin resistance through the activation of inflammatory signaling intermediates that directly may be involved in serine phosphorylation of IRS-1 within insulin sensitive cell types such as skeletal muscle cells, endothelial cells, adicocytes and thereby in inducing insulin resistance.

5. Perspectives

An aspect that can be directly related to insulin resistance and at the same time be involved in the increased cardiovascular morbility and mortality in patients with hypertension could be the lack of cytoprotective effect of the insulin. In fact, a growing body of evidence indicates that insulin acts as survival hormone. This property plays a key role in protection of organs that are mainly constituted by terminally differentiated cells, like heart and brain, in which death of cells induces irreversible damage and at the same time are target organ of hypertension. Actually, cell death by necrosis or apoptosis plays a key role in pathogenesis of pressure overload-induced left ventricular dysfunction [34]. In vitro and in vivo studies have clearly demonstrated that insulin or insulin-stimulated molecular pathways protect cardiac myocytes from ischemia- or oxidative stress-induced apoptosis [35]. Therefore, one aspect that in the future needs be clarified is whether insulin resistance in the heart and in the brain impairs the cytoprotective effect of the hormone. In this case, insulin resistance in hypertensive patients could increase the rate of cardiovascular events or worsen the prognosis by acting with synergic mechanisms that, on the one hand, increases blood pressure, and on the other hand decrease the cytoprotective properties of the hormone. Therefore, understanding the molecular mechanisms which can interfere with the impairment of an antiapoptotic molecular signal may be useful to improve cardiac and cerebral protection in hypertension.

References

[1] J. Olefsky, J.W. Farquhar, G. Reaven, Relationship between fasting plasma insulin level and resistance to insulin-mediated glucose uptake in normal and diabetic subjects, Diabetes 22 (7) (1973) 507–513.

[2] O.G. Kolterman, et al., Mechanisms of insulin resistance in human obesity: evidence for receptor and postreceptor defects, J. Clin. Invest. 65 (6) (1980) 1272–1284.

[3] E. Ferrannini, et al., Insulin resistance in essential hypertension, N. Engl. J. Med. 317 (6) (1987) 350–357.
[4] Executive summary of the third report of the National Cholesterol Education Program (NCEP) expert panel on detection, evaluation, and treatment of high blood cholesterol in adults (Adult Treatment Panel III), Jama 285 (19) (2001) 2486–2497.
[5] G. Paolisso, et al., Insulin resistance and hyperinsulinemia in patients with chronic congestive heart failure, Metabolism 40 (9) (1991) 972–977.
[6] A. Shah, R.P. Shannon, Insulin resistance in dilated cardiomyopathy, Rev. Cardiovasc. Med. 4 (Suppl 6) (2003) S50–S57.
[7] U. Scherrer, et al., Nitric oxide release accounts for insulin's vascular effects in humans, J. Clin. Invest. 94 (6) (1994) 2511–2515.
[8] J. Lee, P.F. Pilch, The insulin receptor: structure, function, and signaling, Am. J. Physiol. 266 (2 Pt 1) (1994) C319–C334.
[9] L.N. Cong, et al., Physiological role of Akt in insulin-stimulated translocation of GLUT4 in transfected rat adipose cells, Mol. Endocrinol. 11 (13) (1997) 1881–1890.
[10] Y.B. Kim, et al., Normal insulin-dependent activation of Akt/protein kinase B, with diminished activation of phosphoinositide 3-kinase, in muscle in type 2 diabetes, J. Clin. Invest. 104 (6) (1999) 733–741.
[11] K. Egawa, et al., Persistent activation of phosphatidylinositol 3-kinase causes insulin resistance due to accelerated insulin-induced insulin receptor substrate-1 degradation in 3T3-L1 adipocytes, Endocrinology 141 (6) (2000) 1930–1935.
[12] B.J. Goldstein, et al., Regulation of the insulin signalling pathway by cellular protein–tyrosine phosphatases, Mol. Cell. Biochem. 182 (1–2) (1998) 91–99.
[13] G.S. Hotamisligil, Mechanisms of TNF-alpha-induced insulin resistance, Exp. Clin. Endocrinol. Diabetes 107 (2) (1999) 119–125.
[14] G. Lembo, et al., Abnormal sympathetic overactivity evoked by insulin in the skeletal muscle of patients with essential hypertension, J. Clin. Invest. 90 (1) (1992) 24–29.
[15] G. Lembo, et al., Insulin modulation of vascular reactivity is already impaired in prehypertensive spontaneously hypertensive rats, Hypertension 26 (2) (1995) 290–293.
[16] H. Abe, et al., Hypertension, hypertriglyceridemia, and impaired endothelium-dependent vascular relaxation in mice lacking insulin receptor substrate-1, J. Clin. Invest. 101 (8) (1998) 1784–1788.
[17] S.B. Wheatcroft, et al., Preserved glucoregulation but attenuation of the vascular actions of insulin in mice heterozygous for knockout of the insulin receptor, Diabetes 53 (10) (2004) 2645–2652.
[18] Z.J. Cheng, et al., Endothelial dysfunction and salt-sensitive hypertension in spontaneously diabetic Goto-Kakizaki rats, Hypertension 37 (2 Part 2) (2001) 433–439.
[19] Y. Ouchi, et al., Augmented contractile function and abnormal Ca2+ handling in the aorta of Zucker obese rats with insulin resistance, Diabetes 45 (Suppl 3) (1996) S55–S58.
[20] C. Morisco, et al., Insulin-stimulated cardiac glucose uptake is impaired in spontaneously hypertensive rats: role of early steps of insulin signalling, J. Hypertens. 18 (4) (2000) 465–473.
[21] G. Mancia, et al., Sympathetic activation in the pathogenesis of hypertension and progression of organ damage, Hypertension 34 (4 Pt 2) (1999) 724–728.
[22] S. Yusuf, et al., Ramipril and the development of diabetes, Jama 286 (15) (2001) 1882–1885.
[23] S. Julius, et al., Outcomes in hypertensive patients at high cardiovascular risk treated with regimens based on valsartan or amlodipine: the VALUE randomised trial, Lancet 363 (9426) (2004) 2022–2031.
[24] A.J. Scheen, DREAM study: prevention of type 2 diabetes with ramipril and/or rosiglitazone in persons with dysglycaemia but no cardiovascular disease, Rev. Med. Liege, Suppl. 61 (10) (2006) 728–732.
[25] J.R. Sowers, Insulin resistance and hypertension, Am. J. Physiol, Heart Circ. Physiol. 286 (5) (2004) H1597–H1602.
[26] Y. Taniyama, et al., Mechanisms of reactive oxygen species-dependent downregulation of insulin receptor substrate-1 by angiotensin II, Arterioscler. Thromb. Vasc. Biol. 25 (6) (2005) 1142–1147.
[27] T. Ogihara, et al., Angiotensin II-induced insulin resistance is associated with enhanced insulin signaling, Hypertension 40 (6) (2002) 872–879.
[28] F. Andreozzi, et al., Angiotensin II impairs the insulin signaling pathway promoting production of nitric oxide by inducing phosphorylation of insulin receptor substrate-1 on Ser312 and Ser616 in human umbilical vein endothelial cells, Circ. Res. 94 (9) (2004) 1211–1218.

[29] J. Klein, et al., Beta(3)-adrenergic stimulation differentially inhibits insulin signaling and decreases insulin-induced glucose uptake in brown adipocytes, J. Biol. Chem. 274 (49) (1999) 34795–34802.
[30] C. Morisco, et al., Akt mediates the cross-talk between beta-adrenergic and insulin receptors in neonatal cardiomyocytes, Circ. Res. 96 (2) (2005) 180–188.
[31] T. Nagoshi, et al., PI3K rescues the detrimental effects of chronic Akt activation in the heart during ischemia/reperfusion injury, J. Clin. Invest. 115 (8) (2005) 2128–2138.
[32] P. Dandona, et al., Insulin suppresses plasma concentration of vascular endothelial growth factor and matrix metalloproteinase-9, Diabetes Care 26 (12) (2003) 3310–3314.
[33] A. Aljada, et al., Insulin inhibits the pro-inflammatory transcription factor early growth response gene-1 (Egr)-1 expression in mononuclear cells (MNC) and reduces plasma tissue factor (TF) and plasminogen activator inhibitor-1 (PAI-1) concentrations, J. Clin. Endocrinol. Metab. 87 (3) (2002) 1419–1422.
[34] G. Condorelli, et al., Increased cardiomyocyte apoptosis and changes in proapoptotic and antiapoptotic genes bax and bcl-2 during left ventricular adaptations to chronic pressure overload in the rat, Circulation 99 (23) (1999) 3071–3078.
[35] A.K. Jonassen, et al., Insulin administered at reoxygenation exerts a cardioprotective effect in myocytes by a possible anti-apoptotic mechanism, J. Mol. Cell. Cardiol. 32 (5) (2000) 757–764.

The Metabolic Syndrome: the significance of microvascular and macrovascular diseases

International Congress Series 1303 (2007) 51–59

ELSEVIER

www.ics-elsevier.com

Diabetic nephropathy: An update on renal structure

Paola Fioretto *, Marino Bruseghin, Isabella Barzon, Marco Arboit, Michele Dalla Vestra

Department of Medical and Surgical Sciences, University of Padova Medical School, via Giustiniani 2, 35128 Padova, Italy

Abstract. The renal lesions underlying renal dysfunction differ in type 1 and type 2 diabetes, although the clinical manifestations of diabetic nephropathy, proteinuria, decreased glomerular filtration rate and increasing blood pressure are similar. Indeed, in type 1 diabetes, although also tubular, interstitial and arteriolar lesions are present, the most important structural changes involve the glomerulus, while several type 2 diabetic patients, despite the presence of microalbuminuria or proteinuria, have normal glomerular structure with or without tubulo-interstitial and arteriolar abnormalities. The clinical manifestations of diabetic nephropathy are strongly related with the structural changes, especially with the degree of mesangial expansion in both type 1 and type 2 diabetes. In the last years it has been demonstrated that also changes in the structure and number of podocytes may be involved in the progression of diabetic nephropathy. Previous studies using light and electron microscopic morphometric analysis described the renal structural changes and the renal structural–functional relationships, documenting the contribution of kidney biopsy studies in understanding the pathogenesis of diabetic nephropathy and in identifying the patients with higher risk to progress to end stage renal disease. Finally this review will summarize studies in pancreas transplant recipients demonstrating that the lesions of diabetic nephropathy in humans are reversible, if normoglycemia is achieved and maintained for a long period of time. © 2007 Published by Elsevier B.V.

Keywords: Diabetic nephropathy; Kidney biopsy; Renal structure

1. Light microscopy

The renal morphologic lesions of diabetic nephropathy in type 1 diabetic patients occur in the glomeruli, the arterioles, the interstitium and the tubules [1–5].

* Corresponding author. Tel.: +39 049 8211879; fax: +39 049 8212151.
E-mail address: paola.fioretto@unipd.it (P. Fioretto).

doi:10.1016/j.ics.2007.03.030

In type 1 diabetes glomerulopathy is the most important lesion, characterized by thickening of glomerular basement membrane (GBM) and mesangial expansion, although also the tubules, interstitium and arterioles undergo substantial changes [1].

GBM thickening, the first measurable change, has been documented as early as 1.5 to 2.5 years after the onset of type 1 diabetes [6,7]. Mesangial expansion develops later; an increase in the matrix component of the mesangium can be detected as early as 5–7 years after the onset of diabetes [8–10]. Thereafter these structural changes do not develop at the same rate in the individual patients [11], however when renal insufficiency occurs, marked mesangial expansion and increased GBM width are present in all type 1 diabetic patients [9,10]. Diffuse and generalized mesangial expansion, commonly termed diffuse diabetic glomerulosclerosis, can be associated with nodular lesions consisting of areas of marked mesangial expansion forming large round fibrillar mesangial zones with palisading of mesangial nuclei around the periphery of the nodule and extreme compression of the associated glomerular capillaries (Kimmelstiel–Wilson nodules). Both mesangial expansion and GBM thickening are consequence of extracellular matrix (ECM) accumulation, with increased deposition of types IV and VI collagen, laminin and fibronectin [12,13]. It is not clear whether these changes are caused by increased production of these glycoproteins, decreased degradation or both.

Additional structural abnormalities include glomerular enlargement, tubular basement membrane (TBM) thickening, tubular atrophy [3], interstitial expansion [4], afferent and efferent arteriolar hyalinosis [5]. Also Bowman's capsule thickening is regularly present.

Afferent and efferent arteriolar hyalinosis occurs few years after the onset of diabetes [5]. This is an exudative lesion, mainly due to the replacement of the smooth muscle cells by plasma proteins, especially immunoglobulins, complement, fibrinogen and albumin. The severity of arteriolar hyalinosis is significantly correlated with percent sclerosed glomeruli [5], suggesting that this vascular lesion could contribute to global glomerular sclerosis through severe compromise of glomerular blood flow. Similar lesions are sometimes present also in the glomerular subendothelial space (hyaline caps) and along the parietal surface of Bowman's capsule (capsular drops).

Recently Najafian et al. [14] explored the glomerulotubular junction in proteinuric type 1 diabetic patients. Glomerulotubular junctions were classified as: normal tubules (NT), atrophic tubules (AT) with flattened epithelium, lacking brush borders or no epithelium in association with TBM, or atubular glomeruli (AG) when no tubular connection was observed. AT were subcategorized in short atrophic tubules (SAT), characterized by tubular atrophy at the beginning of proximal tubule, long atrophic tubules (LAT) with tubular atrophy over a longer segment of proximal tubule and atrophic tubules with no observable glomerular opening (ATNO) i.e. with no observable connection between glomerular urinary space and proximal tubular lumen. Atubular glomeruli have open circulation, but no observable tubular attachment and are presumably non functioning. Seventeen percent of glomeruli were atubular and 51% were attached to atrophic tubules. These abnormalities in the glomerulartubular junction were often associated with tip lesions, consisting of dilated capillary loops close to the glomerulotubular junction, with or without mesangiolysis, sometimes filled with foamy cells or PAS-positive hyaline material, with adhesion to Bowman's capsule. Interestingly the lesions at the glomerulotubular junction were strongly related to glomerular filtration rate (GFR) [14]; thus these lesions should be added to the well known constellation of lesions, described above, contributing to the loss of renal function in type 1 diabetes. Whether changes occurring in this crucial area of the nephron occur in the early stages of diabetic nephropathy is unknown.

In type 2 diabetes the situation is more complex. Parving et al.[15] described a high prevalence of non diabetic glomerular diseases in Danish type 2 diabetic patients with proteinuria, with 23% of the patients having a variety of glomerulopathies including minimal lesion nephropathy, chronic glomerulonephritis, and mesangial proliferative glomerulonephritis alone or superimposed to diabetic structural abnormalities. Lipkin [16] described that only 50 of 82 type 2 diabetic patients with nephropathy had typical diabetic glomerulopathy; similarly Gambara et al.[17] found that 33% of proteinuric type 2 diabetic patients had glomerular disease superimposed on diabetic glomerulosclerosis, although more recently the same group reported that non diabetic glomerulopathies occurred only in 18% of type 2 diabetic patients with proteinuria [18]. In the study of Olsen [19] only 12% of the proteinuric patients had non diabetic renal diseases. Therefore the real frequency of non diabetic renal diseases among patients with type 2 diabetes and proteinuria is difficult to asses, and the broad variability is likely to be related to the different biopsy policies adopted, as recently discussed by Mazzucco et al. [20].

We studied a large cohort of type 2 diabetic patients with microalbuminuria and proteinuria and described heterogeneity in renal structure among these patients: in fact only a subset had diabetic glomerulopathy, while the remaining had mild or absent glomerulopathy with or without tubulo-interstitial and arteriolar changes [21]. In our proteinuric patients less than 10% had non diabetic renal diseases.

Thus we proposed a classification system which included 3 major groups [21]:

- Category C I: Normal or near normal renal structure. These patients (35% of microalbuminuric patients (MA) and 15% of proteinuric patients (P)) had biopsies which were normal or showed very mild glomerular, tubular, interstitial and vascular changes.
- Category C II: Typical diabetic nephropathology. These patients (30% of MA and 50% of P) had established diabetic lesions with an approximately balanced severity of glomerular, tubulo-interstitial and arteriolar changes. This picture is typical of that seen in type 1 diabetic patients with obvious light microscopic diabetic nephropathy changes.
- Category C III: Atypical patterns of renal injury. These patients (35% of MA and P) had relatively mild diabetic glomerular changes considering the disproportionately severe renal structural changes including: (a) Tubular atrophy, tubular basement membrane thickening and reduplication and interstitial fibrosis (tubulo-interstitial lesions). (b) Advanced glomerular arteriolar hyalinosis commonly associated with atherosclerosis of larger vessels. (c) Global glomerular sclerosis. In C III group these patterns were present in all possible combinations.

Thus hyperglycaemia may cause different patterns of renal injury in type 2 compared to type 1 diabetic patients. The tubulo-interstitial and vascular changes could also be related to aging, atherosclerosis and systemic hypertension. However, hypertension was present in almost all patients in all 3 structural categories, and "per se" cannot account for the different lesions observed in Category C III. Further, mean age was similar in the patients in Category C II and C III (60 years), despite the different patterns of renal injury in the two groups, and our observations in a large number of age-matched normal controls argue that aging is not sufficient to explain most of the renal structural changes observed in C III patients. Thus it can be hypothesized that the heterogeneity in renal structure might reflect the heterogeneous nature of type 2 diabetes.

2. Electron microscopic studies and structural–functional relationships

The relationships between structural abnormalities and kidney function are better defined using electron microscopic morphometric analysis. The critical lesion in type 1 diabetes is mesangial expansion, morphometrically termed mesangial fractional volume [Vv(mes/glom)] (the percentage of the cross-sectional area of the glomerular tuft made up by mesangium); this is the structural parameter that best correlates with all functional parameters in type 1 diabetes [9,22]. Indeed a highly significant inverse correlation exists between Vv(mes/glom) and GFR [9]; when mesangium expands it restricts and distorts glomerular capillaries and diminishes capillary filtration surface, which is strongly inversely related to Vv(mes/glom) and directly to GFR [23]. Vv(mes/glom) is also related to albumin excretion rate (AER) and blood pressure levels [24]. In contrast GBM thickening is not related to GFR or to the presence of hypertension, but only to AER, suggesting that this lesion is involved in the pathogenesis of albuminuria, rather than in the loss of kidney function. Also interstitial expansion and percentage of global sclerosis are related to proteinuria, hypertension and declining GFR [4,5]. In the early stages of diabetic nephropathy, however, our data in a small number of patients with type 1 diabetes studied with sequential renal biopsies, indicate that progression from normoalbuminuria to microalbuminuria and from microalbuminuria to early overt nephropathy is related only to progressive mesangial expansion [11]; in contrast there was no progression in interstitial fibrosis or GBM thickening. These data are partially in contrast with a recent study describing that GBM width at baseline biopsy was predictive of AER after six years of follow-up [25].

Mesangial expansion and interstitial expansion are independent determinants of renal dysfunction in type 1 diabetes and are probably consequence of different pathogenetic mechanisms. Indeed mesangial expansion is mainly due to ECM accumulation; in contrast early interstitial expansion is due to an increase of the cellular component, whereas the increase of interstitial collagen occurs only in patients with advanced diabetic nephropathy [26]. Thus in type 1 diabetes clinical nephropathy is always associated with advanced glomerular injury.

In the early stages of the disease, we have studied glomerular structure in four groups of type 1 diabetic patients with increasing levels of AER, ranging from normoalbuminuria to high levels of microalbuminuria. All parameters of glomerulopathy were abnormal in the normoalbuminuric group, although approximately half of the patients fell into the normal range. No patients with AER >30 μg/min had GBM width and Vv(mes/glom) in the normal range [8]. Interestingly in several normoalbuminuric patients Vv(mes/glom) and GBM width overlapped with the values in patients with high levels of microalbuminuria [8]. It is tempting to hypothesize that normoalbuminuric patients with established lesions have an increased risk to progress to microalbuminuria and proteinuria and that those patients with increased AER, but glomerular parameters near the normal range may revert to normoalbuminuria. This hypothesis has recently been reinforced by a study suggesting that in long-standing normoalbuminuric type 1 diabetic patients glomerular structure is predictive of the course of renal function over the time [27].

In type 2 diabetes our findings indicate that mesangial expansion is also a crucial structural change, leading to loss of renal function; AER was directly related to both GBM width (r=0.47) and Vv(mes/glom) (r=0.44), but GFR was inversely related only to Vv (mes/glom) (r=0.47) and not to GBM width [28]. Although these structural–functional relationships were significant, they were imprecise and less strong than in type 1 diabetes. Moreover, confirming our observations from light microscopic studies [21], glomerular lesions were less advanced in type 2 than type 1 diabetic patients and a substantial number of these patients had normal glomerular structure despite abnormal albumin excretion rate. These data are in agreement with those in Pima Indians, where global glomerular sclerosis, Vv(interstitium) and GBM width were similar in patients with long-term type 2 diabetes with normoalbuminuria and those with microalbuminuria; only Vv(mes/glom) increased from early diabetes to microalbuminuria. In these patients ultrastructural glomerular parameters were significantly abnormal only in patients with clinical nephropathy [29].

Hayashi et al. [30] reported in type 2 diabetic patients renal structural–functional relationships similar to those observed in type 1 diabetes. In contrast Østerby et al. [31] described great variability in glomerular injury in Danish type 2 diabetic patients with proteinuria; they also outlined that type 2 diabetic patients tended to have less marked glomerular changes than type 1 with comparable renal function.

Of prognostic relevance, the heterogeneity in renal structure is related to the risk of progressive GFR loss [32]. Indeed GFR decline over 4 years of follow-up in type 2 diabetic patients with microalbuminuria and proteinuria was significantly correlated with the severity of mesangial expansion and GBM thickening [32].

3. Role of podocytes in diabetic nephropathy

Podocytes are injured in numerous experimental and human glomerular diseases, including minimal-change disease, focal segmental glomerulosclerosis, collapsing glomerulopathy, lupus nephritis and diabetic nephropathy [33,34].

The understanding of the role of podocytes in diabetic nephropathy is increasing in recent years, although definitive conclusions have not been reached. White et al. [35] observed similar numbers of podocytes in normal subjects and in type 1 diabetic patients with abnormal albumin excretion rate although there was a trend towards fewer podocytes per glomerulus in diabetic patients. Moreover, this study found no significant correlation between podocyte number and AER. These findings are in contrast with a previous study [36] reporting that podocyte number was decreased in type 1 diabetic patients with normal albumin excretion rate, when compared to normal controls, suggesting that diabetes per se may affect podocytes. Bjorn et al. [37] described an increase of foot process width on the peripheral GBM in type 1 diabetic patients with abnormal albumin excretion rate compared with normoalbuminuric patients, without significant differences between microalbuminurics and proteinurics. In contrast, Ellis et al.[38] found that podocyte structure was significantly altered only in patients with type 1 diabetes and overt proteinuria and that there was no difference between patients with microalbuminuria and patients with normal albumin excretion rate for foot process width and filtration slit length density; however, when all diabetic patients were considered these parameters were correlated with AER. Low podocyte number has been described also in type 2 diabetic Pima Indians with proteinuria [29]. In these patients podocyte loss and increased foot process width have been suggested to play a role in the progression to overt nephropathy. This concept was reinforced in a recent longitudinal study, where Pima Indians with type 2 diabetes and microalbuminuria were studied during a 4 years follow-up [39]; the number of podocytes per glomerulus at baseline was the strongest predictor of the changes in albuminuria in that patients with the lowest number of podocytes had the highest risk of fast progression to overt proteinuria [39]. We studied podocyte structure in a large cohort of Caucasian type 2 diabetic patients, with AER ranging from normal to overt proteinuria [40]. The density of podocytes per glomerulus [Nv(epi/glom)] was significantly decreased in all diabetic patients compared to controls, and was lower in microalbuminuric and proteinuric patients than in normoalbuminuric. The absolute number of podocytes per glomerulus (Epi N/glom) was lower in microalbuminuric and proteinuric patients compared to controls; however there were no significant differences among the diabetic groups. In addition microalbuminuric and proteinuric patients had decreased length density of filtration slits over the peripheral GBM (FSLv/glom), and increased foot process width (FPW) compared to normoalbuminuric. AER was inversely related to Nv(epi/glom) and FSLv/glom and directly to FPW, while there was no correlation with Epi N/glom. GFR was weakly related only to FSLv/glom. Since several patients with abnormal AER had normal Vv(mes/glom) (≤ 0.25) we compared their podocyte structure to that of normoalbuminurics with normal Vv(mes/glom). Patients with abnormal AER had lower Nv(epi/glom) and FSLv/glom and higher FPW than normoalbuminurics. These results suggest that in Caucasian type 2 diabetic patients changes in podocyte structure and density occur since the early stages of diabetic nephropathy and might contribute to increasing albuminuria in these patients. Moreover, podocyte structural changes could in part explain abnormal albuminuria in patients without diabetic glomerulopathy. These findings also suggest that in type 2 diabetic patients the density of podocytes may be functionally more relevant than the absolute number [40].

Podocytes have limited capacity to replicate and when they are lost they cannot be replaced by new cells; thus it has been hypothesized that the loss of podocytes, along with the increase in glomerular volume, caused by diabetes, necessarily require the residual cells to cover a larger area of GBM. This could cause foot process widening and reduce the ability of the podocytes to remain attached to GBM, forming areas of bare GBM with consequent proteinuria. Moreover these areas are potential starting points for glomerular sclerosis.

Indeed studies in rats [41] with reduced nephron number and consequent glomerular hypertrophy have demonstrated that podocytes suffer progressive injury when forced to cover a larger surface area. Initially these rats develop proteinuria and foot process widening, and subsequently glomerular sclerosis.

Further studies on podocyte ultrastructure and on the expression of slit diaphragm proteins (nephrin, podocin, P-cadherin etc) are necessary to better define the role of these cells in the pathogenesis of diabetic nephropathy.

4. Reversibility of diabetic nephropathy lesions

Pancreas transplantation offers the opportunity to test the capability of long-term normoglycemia to prevent, halt or reverse diabetic nephropathy lesions. Pancreas transplantation, performed in uremic patients at the time of renal transplant or, less frequently, after kidney transplant, prevents or slows the development of early diabetic glomerulopathy lesions in the renal allograft [42–44].

The possibility of reversal can be addressed by studying long-term non uremic type 1 diabetic recipients of pancreas transplantation alone (PTA). We have studied 13 PTA recipients and found that, despite 5 years of normoglycemia, there was no amelioration of the lesions of diabetic nephropathy [45]. GBM width was abnormal before PTA in these patients and was unchanged after 5 years. Vv(Mes/glom) was increased compared to the baseline biopsies, due to a decrease in glomerular volume (GV), while the total mesangial volume per glomerulus remained unchanged [45]. Eight of the 13 PTA recipients were available for studies after 10 years of normoglycemia [46]. These patients were 33±3 (mean±S.D.) years old, had a duration of diabetes of 22±5 years, and an HbA1c of 8.7±1.5% at the time of PTA. GFR was significantly decreased (by 30%) at 5 years post PTA and did not change thereafter. Albumin excretion rate tended to decrease at 10 years, although not significantly. The data on renal function in these patients are, however, complex to interpret, given the confounding effects of cyclosporine. Indeed there was a significant correlation between the changes in GFR and cyclosporine dose and blood levels in these patients, especially in the post-transplant first year [47]. There was, as already noted, no beneficial effects on glomerular structure at 5 years post-PTA, while obvious reversal of diabetic glomerular and tubular lesions was observed in all 8 patients 10 years after PTA [46]. Thus, GBM and TBM widths, unchanged at 5 years, decreased at 10-year follow-up, returning to normal values in most patients. Vv(Mes/glom) and mesangial matrix fractional volume (Vv(MM/glom) which had increased from baseline to 5 years, were lower at 10 years than at baseline or 5 years. Light microscopic observations revealed a remarkable amelioration of glomerular structure in these patients, including the total disappearance of Kimmelstiel–Wilson nodular lesions and reopening of glomerular capillaries previously compressed by mesangial expansion. We observed also remodelling of the tubulo-interstitial lesions, with decrease in the 10 years biopsies of cortical interstitial fractional volume, the fractional volume of tubules which were atrophic and an overall decrease in renal interstitial fibrillar collagen [48]. The reasons for the long delay in reversal of diabetic nephropathy lesions are unknown; nevertheless the long time necessary for these diabetic lesions to disappear is consistent with their slow development. In fact, diabetic renal lesions develop and progress from onset of diabetes over at least one decade before they can cause any functional abnormality. Regardless of the mechanisms involved, at some point after PTA, glomerular, tubular and interstitial cells changed their behaviour towards ECM removal and architectural remodelling in remarkable demonstrations of the recooperative capacity of the kidney.

These findings call for further studies aimed at identifying the molecular and cellular mechanisms involved in these healing processes could provide new directions in the treatment of DN.

References

[1] M. Mauer, et al., Diabetic nephropathy, in: R.W. Schrier (Ed.), Disease of the Kidney and Urinary Tract, Lippincott Williams and Wilkins, Philadelphia, 2001, pp. 2083–2127.

[2] E.T. Bell, Renal vascular disease in diabetes mellitus, Diabetes 2 (1953) 376–389.

[3] P. Brito, et al., Proximal tubular basement membrane width in insulin-dependent diabetes mellitus, Kidney Int. 53 (1998) 754–761.

[4] P.H. Lane, et al., Renal interstitial expansion in insulin-dependent diabetes mellitus, Kidney Int. 43 (1993) 661–667.
[5] R.D. Harris, et al., Global glomerular sclerosis and glomerular arteriolar hyalinosis in insulin-dependent diabetes, Kidney Int. 40 (1991) 107–114.
[6] R. Østerby, Early phases in the development of diabetic glomerulopathy, Acta Med. Scand. 475 (1975) 1–7.
[7] R. Østerby, Morphometric studies of the peripheral glomerular basement membrane in early juvenile diabetes I. Development of initial basement membrane thickening, Diabetologia 8 (1972) 84–92.
[8] P. Fioretto, M.W. Steffes, S.M. Mauer, Glomerular structure in non-proteinuric insulin-dependent diabetic patients with various levels of albuminuria, Diabetes 43 (1994) 1358–1364.
[9] S.M. Mauer, et al., Structural functional relationships in diabetic nephropathy, J. Clin. Invest. 74 (1984) 1143–1155.
[10] R. Osterby, A.R. Andersen, H.J. Gundersen, Quantitative studies of glomerular ultrastructure in type 1 diabetics with incipient nephropathy, Diabet. Nephropathy 3 (1984) 95.
[11] P. Fioretto, et al., Sequential renal biopsies in IDDM patients: structural factors associated with clinical progression, Kidney Int. 48 (1995) 1929–1935.
[12] R.J. Falk, et al., Polyantigenic expansion of basement membrane constituents in diabetic nephropathy, Diabetes 32 (1983) 34.
[13] Y. Kim, et al., Differential expression of basement membrane collagen chains in diabetic nephropathy, Am. J. Pathol. 138 (1991) 413.
[14] B. Najafian, et al., Atubular glomeruli and glomerulotubular junction abnormalities in diabetic nephropathy, J. Am. Soc. Nephrol. 14 (2003) 908–917.
[15] H.H. Parving, et al., Prevalence and causes of albuminuria in non-insulin-dependent diabetic patients, Kidney Int. 41 (1992) 758–762.
[16] G.W. Lipkin, More than one kind of type 2 diabetes with renal disease do not have diabetic nephropathy, J. Am. Soc. Nephrol. 5 (1994) 37.
[17] V. Gambara, et al., Heterogeneous nature of renal lesions in type II diabetes, J. Am. Soc. Nephrol. 3 (1993) 1458–1466.
[18] P. Ruggenenti, et al., The nephropathy of non insulin dependent diabetes: predictors of outcome relative to diverse patters of renal injury, J. Am. Soc. Nephrol. 9 (1998) 2336–2343.
[19] S. Olsen, C.E. Mogensen, Non-diabetic renal disease in NIDDM proteinuric patients may be rare in biopsies from clinical practice, Diabetologia 39 (1996) 1638–1645.
[20] G. Mazzucco, T. Bertani, M. Fortunato, Different patterns of renal damage in type 2 diabetes mellitus: a multicentric study on 393 biopsies, Am. J. Kidney Dis. 39 (2002) 713–720.
[21] P. Fioretto, et al., Patterns of renal injury in type 2 (non insulin dependent) diabetic patients with microalbuminuria, Diabetologia 39 (1996) 1569–1576.
[22] B.M. Chavers, et al., Glomerular lesions and urinary albumin excretion rate in type 1 diabetic patients without overt proteinuria, N. Engl. J. Med. 320 (1989) 966–970.
[23] E.N. Ellis, et al., Glomerular filtration surface in type 1 diabetes mellitus, Kidney Int. 29 (1986) 889.
[24] S.M. Mauer, D.E.R. Sutherland, M.W. Steffes, Relationships of systemic blood pressure to nephropathy in insulin-dependent diabetes mellitus, Kidney Int. 41 (1992) 736.
[25] H.J. Bangstad, et al., Severity of glomerulopathy predicts long-term urinary albumin excretion rate in patients with type 1 diabetes and microalbuminuria, Diabetes Care 22 (1999) 314–319.
[26] A. Katz, et al., An increase in the cell component of the cortical interstitium antedates interstitial fibrosis in type 1 diabetic patients, Kidney Int. 61 (2002) 2058–2066.
[27] M.L. Caramori, P. Fioretto, M. Mauer, Low glomerular filtration rate in normoalbuminuric type 1 diabetic patients: an indicator of more advanced glomerular lesions, Diabetes 52 (2003) 1036–1040.
[28] P. Fioretto, et al., Glomerular ultrastructure in type 2 diabetes, J. Am. Soc. Nephrol. 9 (1998) 114 A (Abs).
[29] M.E. Pagtalunan, et al., Podocyte loss and progressive glomerular injury in type 2 diabetes, J. Clin. Invest. 99 (1997) 342–348.
[30] H. Hayashi, et al., An electron microscopic study of glomeruli in Japanese patients with non-insulin dependent diabetes mellitus, Kidney Int. 41 (1992) 749–757.
[31] R. Østerby, et al., Glomerular structure and function in proteinuric type 2 (non insulin dependent) diabetic patients, Diabetologia 36 (1993) 1064–1070.

[32] R. Nosadini, et al., Course of renal function in type 2 diabetic patients with abnormalities of albumin excretion rate, Diabetes 49 (2000) 476–484.
[33] L. Barisoni, P. Mundel, Podocyte biology and the emerging understanding of podocyte diseases, Am. J. Nephrol. 23 (2003) 353–360.
[34] W. Kriz, N. Gretz, K.V. Lemley, Progression of glomerular disease: is the podocyte the culprit? Kidney Int. 54 (1998) 687–697.
[35] K.E. White, et al., Podocyte number in normotensive type 1 diabetic patients with albuminuria, Diabetes 51 (2002) 3083–3089.
[36] M.W. Steffes, et al., Glomerular cell number in normal subjects and in type 1 diabetic patients, Kidney Int. 59 (2001) 2104–2113.
[37] S.F. Bjorn, et al., Glomerular epithelial foot process and filtration slits in IDDM patients, Diabetologia 38 (1995) 1197–1204.
[38] E.N. Ellis, et al., Observation of glomerular epithelial cell structure in patients with type I diabetes mellitus, Kidney Int. 32 (1987) 736–741.
[39] T.W. Meyer, P.H. Bennett, R.G. Nelson, Podocyte number predicts long-term urinary albumin excretion in Pima Indians with Type II diabetes and microalbuminuria, Diabetologia 42 (1999) 1341–1344 (2).
[40] M. Dalla Vestra, et al., Is podocyte injury relevant in diabetic nephropathy? Studies in patients with type 2 diabetes, Diabetes 52 (2003) 1031–1035.
[41] J.W.U. Fries, et al., Glomerular hypertrophy and epithelial cell injury modulate progressive glomerulosclerosis in the rat, Lab. Invest. 60 (1989) 205–218.
[42] S.O. Bohman, et al., Prevention of kidney graft diabetic nephropathy by pancreas transplantation in man, Diabetes 34 (1985) 306–308.
[43] H.E. Wilczek, et al., Pancreatic graft protects a simultaneously transplanted kidney from developing diabetic nephropathy: a 1 to 6 year follow-up study, Transplant. Proc. 1 (1993) 1314–1315.
[44] R.W. Bilous, et al., The effects of pancreas transplantation on the glomerular structure of renal allografts in patients with insulin-dependent diabetes, N. Engl. J. Med. 32 (1989) 80–85.
[45] P. Fioretto, et al., Effects of pancreas transplantation on glomerular structure in insulin-dependent diabetic patients with their own kidneys, Lancet 342 (1993) 1193–1196.
[46] P. Fioretto, et al., Reversal of lesions of diabetic nephropathy after pancreas transplantation, N. Engl. J. Med. 339 (1998) 69–75.
[47] P. Fioretto, et al., Cyclosporine associated lesions in native kidneys of diabetic pancreas transplant recipients, Kidney Int. 48 (1995) 489–495.
[48] P. Fioretto, et al., Remodeling of renal interstitial and tubular lesions in pancreas transplant at recipients, Kidney Int. 69 (2006) 907–912.

ELSEVIER

International Congress Series 1303 (2007) 60–64

www.ics-elsevier.com

Erectile dysfunction as a predictor of cardiovascular risk

Piero Montorsi *

Institute of Cardiology, University of Milan, Centro Cardiologico Monzino, IRCCS, Milan, Italy

Abstract. Evidence is accumulating in favour of a link between erectile dysfunction (ED) and coronary artery disease (CAD). Prevalence of common risk factors for atherosclerosis is similar. ED is frequently found in patients with CAD and shares a similar pathogenic involvement of nitric oxide-pathway leading to impairment of endothelium-dependent vasodilatation (early phase) and structural vascular abnormalities (late phase). Moreover, there is room to consider ED as a marker of early sub-clinical CAD. It is therefore crucial to identify asymptomatic patients with ED who may be at risk of occult CAD. Initial screening may adopt risk assessment office-based approaches to score patient into low, intermediate or high risk of future cardiovascular events. Attention should be drawn to patients at intermediate risk. Targets for the assessment of sub-clinical CAD in this subset of patients should include both obstructive and non-obstructive CAD. Although less investigated, non-obstructive CAD is a more important target to assess since acute myocardial infarction is the result of an acute occlusion of a previously non critical coronary vessel. Several non-invasive tests may add important diagnostic and prognostic information in patients at intermediate coronary risk. Some of these directly assess coronary atherosclerosis burden – such as coronary calcium score by electron beam computed tomography – whereas others, such as carotid intima-media thickness by ultrasound are surrogates of coronary involvement.

Keywords: Erectile dysfunction; Cardiovascular risk; Acute coronary events

Erectile dysfunction (ED) is defined as the inability to reach or maintain erection sufficient for satisfactory sexual performance. Evidence is accumulating in favour of ED as a vascular disorder in the majority of patients. Common risk factors for atherosclerosis are prevalent in patients with ED and the extent of ED has been related to the number and severity of risk factors themselves [1,2]. Besides, the prevalence of ED is increased in patients with

* Tel.: +39 02 58002576; fax: +39 02 58002398.
E-mail address: piero.montorsi@unimi.it.

0531-5131/
doi:10.1016/j.ics.2007.03.021

vascular diseases such as coronary artery disease (CAD) [3–5], diabetes [2,6], cerebrovascular disease [7], hypertension and peripheral arterial disease [8,9]. Finally, ED and vascular diseases share a similar pathogenic involvement of nitric oxide pathway leading to impairment of endothelium-dependent vasodilatation (early phase) and structural vascular abnormalities (late phase) [10–12]. Thus, ED may be considered as the clinical manifestation of a vascular disease affecting penile circulation likewise angina pectoris is the clinical manifestation of a vascular disorder affecting coronary circulation. Moreover, there is growing evidence that ED may be an early sign of a systemic, largely sub-clinical vascular atherosclerotic involvement, mainly at the level of coronary circulation (i.e. ED as "sentinel of the heart").

1. ED as a marker of early CAD: the artery size hypothesis

To explain the temporal relationship between penile and coronary circulation we proposed a pathophysiological mechanism, named the "artery size" hypothesis [13–15], based on the conceptual model that exposure to common risk factors leads sequentially and uniformly across all vascular beds to endothelial dysfunction, intima-media thickening and, lately, vascular obstruction and flow-limiting stenoses. The reason why symptoms rarely become clinically evident in different arterial districts at the same time in a given patient may be the result of larger vessels (i.e. coronary arteries) being able to better tolerate the same amount of plaque as compared to smaller ones (i.e. penile arteries) without inducing flow-limiting stenosis. According to this putative mechanism, ED and CAD should be considered as two different aspects of the same disease, with an expected temporal relationship (i.e. ED should become manifest earlier than CAD). Consequently, men with ED as the first complain should rarely complain of significant CAD whereas men with overt CAD should frequently suffer concomitant ED.

Several reports have been published supporting this hypothesis. Kaiser et al. [16] first reported on the role of ED as a very early marker of "cardiovascular disease". They compared a small group of patients with no risk factors and ED ($n=30$) since at least 6 months with an age-matched control group without ED ($n=27$). All patients were submitted to a throughout cardiovascular work-up that included flow-mediated brachial artery vasodilation by Doppler ultrasound (as an index of endothelial function), carotid intima-media thickness and coronary calcium score by multislice computed tomography. It was found that ED patients had a significantly reduced vasodilator response to occlusion test (1.3 ± 0.3 vs. $2.4 \pm 0.3\%$, $p=0.014$) as the only abnormal CV test compared to controls. This finding confirmed that endothelial dysfunction is the early alteration of ED that is detectable well before the development of common vascular abnormalities. Similarly, Bocchio et al. [17] investigated biochemical measures (sP selectin, sICAM-1, sVCAM-1 and endothelin-1) of endothelial cell activation in ED patients without common risk factors and in healthy age-matched controls. They found that increased endothelin-1 was the best independent predictor for ED (OR 5.37, CI: 2.12–19.70) after being adjusted for the confounding effect of BMI and smoking.

We tested the "artery size hypothesis" in 300 consecutive unselected patients with angiographically documented CAD [4]. ED was detected by the international index of erectile function questionnaire in 149/300 (49%). Among those with ED, 67% reported that sexual symptoms preceded anginal symptoms by a mean interval of 34 months (range 1–168). A recent study from our institution in a more selected patient population with CAD (patients with chronic angina pectoris) confirmed the initial observation and showed that virtually all patients (93%) had ED symptoms before angina pectoris onset, with a mean interval of 24 [12–36] months [18].

2. ED as predictor of future cardiovascular events: clinical evidence

The issue whether patients with ED do have a higher long-term risk of cardiovascular events as compared to general population without ED is yet to be resolved. A well planned prospective study is still lacking. Available data come primarily from retrospective investigations. One of these reviews examined 2.115 men with several risk factors at a large primary care clinic [19]. Those who had ED when first seen were 3 times more likely to have AMI in the past. By contrast, the overall association between ED and subsequent AMI was greater (OR: 4.9, CI 1.9–12.7) but lost statistical significance when adjusted for age (OR: 2.2, CI 0.7–6.6) in part due to the small number of events (17/1844) in the 2 year-F/U. Blumentals et al. [20] examined a large cohort of patients ($n=12.825$) with diagnosis of ED recruited by an administrative database compared with a similar number of controls without ED. The ED group had a two-fold increase (OR: 1.99, CI 1.17–3.38) in the risk of AMI as compared to non-ED patients after adjusting for age at ED diagnosis, smoking, obesity, use of medications such as ace-inhibitors, beta-blockers and statins. Study limitations were mainly inherent to the type of database used that included only patients with established ED and AMI (probably the most severe cases), and lack information about potential co-morbidity and diabetes. Conversely, Ströberg et al. [21], sent a questionnaire about sexual function to 160 patients who suffered AMI 2 years before. Among 100 who responded (mean age 59 years), ED prevalence was 34%, duration was <3 years in the majority and score was severe in $<10\%$. Interestingly, control group of similar age without previous AMI had an ED rate of 30%, raising doubts about ED as predictive marker of acute coronary syndromes.

Finally, a very recent paper by Thompson et al. [22] made a substantial step forward in this issue. Among 9457 subjects enrolling in the Prostate Cancer Prevention Trial (finasteride vs. placebo), 4247 had no sexual dysfunction at study entry and represent the study cohort of patients. They were followed up every 3 months for 5 years looking at the onset of ED and cardiovascular events. Fifty-seven percent of subjects developed ED over the time. After adjusting for all covariates, men with incident ED had a significantly increased risk of acute myocardial infarction or angina as compared to those without incident ED (HR: 1.37; CI: 1.06–1.76, $p=0.02$). ED had an equal or greater effect on subsequent CV events of the same magnitude as family history of premature coronary artery disease (CAD), smoking or hypercholesterolemia.

3. ED as a marker of sub-clinical CAD: which patient should be screened?

Given the high prevalence of ED in middle-aged population and its clinical significance, a systematic cardiologic screening would be not cost-effective. Therefore, it is crucial to identify ED patients at high risk for occult CAD and/or acute coronary events. A reasonable first step is to estimate, through one of many risk assessment office-based approaches, the subject's own relative and absolute risk of cardiovascular event (usually in the following 10 years). Although none of these tools is yet considered ideal, the Framingham Risk Score [23] and the European

System Coronary Risk Evaluation (SCORE) [24] are popular and widely used in US and European countries, respectively. The recently released Second Princeton Consensus Conference recommendations addressed this topic more specifically in patients with sexual dysfunction and heart diseases [16]. According to the presence and/or severity of conventional risk factors subjects are divided into categories at different risk: low (<10%), intermediate (10–20%) and high (>20%). Low-risk patients should be reassured and retested in about 5 years. Medications for ED can be prescribed without need for additional tests. High risk patients – defined as those with overt CAD, diabetes, extra-cardiac atherosclerosis (peripheral arterial disease, symptomatic carotid stenosis, abdominal aortic aneurysm) or asymptomatic subjects with multiple risk factors conferring a 10-year risk of CAD>20% – should undergo further cardiological assessment and should receive aggressive risk factors treatment. In this group of patients, treatment for ED should be deferred until a full cardiologic assessment is performed. Subjects at intermediate risk – representing almost 40% of the US population – may benefit from additional non-invasive tests aimed to better define the presence and the extension of sub-clinical coronary atherosclerosis [25,26]. Some tests address obstructive atherosclerosis by directly assessing coronary flow reserve (i.e. standard exercise stress test, rest/stress myocardial scintigraphy or echocardiography). Other tests are general measures of atherosclerosis burden (not necessarily obstructive) either in the coronary circulation (i.e. coronary calcium score by electron beam computed tomography [EBCT]), or in extra-coronary vessels (i.e. ankle brachial index, carotid intima-media thickness (IMT) by B-mode ultrasound) as surrogate markers of CAD [27,28]. Although a systematic use of these measures of non-obstructive atherosclerosis burden has not been yet recommended in the guidelines for coronary risk assessment, their utilization is progressively being extended from the research area to clinical practice.

References

[1] H.A. Feldman, et al., Impotence and its medical and psychological correlates: results of the Massachusset Male Aging Study, J. Urol. 151 (1994) 54–61.

[2] A. Bortolotti, et al., The epidemiology of erectile dysfunction and its risk factors, Int. J. Androl. 20 (1997) 323–334.

[3] H. Solomon, et al., Relation of erectile dysfunction to angiographic artery disease, Am. J. Cardiol. 91 (2002) 230–231.

[4] F. Montorsi, et al., Erectile dysfunction prevalence, time of onset and association with risk factors in 300 consecutive patients with acute chest pain and angiographically documented coronary artery disease, Eur. Urol. 44 (2003) 360–365.

[5] R. Kloner, et al., Erectile dysfunction in the cardiac patient: how common and should we treat? J. Urol. 170 (2003) S46–S50.

[6] C. Gazzarusso, et al., Relationship between erectile dysfunction and silent myocardial ischemia in apparently uncomplicated type 2 diabetic patients, Circulation 110 (2004) 22–26.

[7] J.T. Korpelainenl, et al., Sexual dysfunction in stoke patients, Acta Neurol. Scand. 98 (1998) 400–405.

[8] M. Burchard, et al., Erectile dysfunction is a marker for cardiovascular complications and psychological functioning in men with hypertension, Int. J. Impot. Res. 13 (2001) 276–281.

[9] R. Virag, P. Bouilly, Is impotence an arterial disease? A study of arterial risk factors in 440 impotence men, Lancet 322 (1985) 181–184.

[10] K.M. Azadzoi, I. Goldstein, Erectile dysfunction due to atherosclerotic vascular disease: the development of a animal model, J. Urol. 147 (1992) 1675–1681.

[11] K.M. Azadzoi, I.S. deTeiada, Hypercholesterolemia impairs endothelium-dependent relaxation of rabbit corpus cavernosum smooth muscle, J. Urol. 146 (1991) 238–240.

[12] H. Solomon, J.W. Man, G. Jackson, Erectile dysfunction and the cardiovascular patient: endothelial dysfunction is the common denominator, Heart 89 (2003) 179–184.
[13] P. Montorsi, F. Montorsi, C. Schulman, Is erectile dysfunction the tip of the iceberg of a systemic vascular disorder? Eur. Urol. 44 (2003) 352–354.
[14] P. Montorsi, et al., The artery size hypothesis: a macrovascular link between erectile dysfunction and coronary artery disease, Am. J. Cardiol. 96 (Suppl) (2005) 19M–23M.
[15] P. Montorsi, et al., Association between erectile dysfunction and coronary artery disease: a case report study, J. Sex Med. 2 (2005) 575–582.
[16] D.R. Kaiser, et al., Impaired brachial artery endothelium-dependent and -independent vasodilation in men with erectile dysfunction and no other clinical cardiovascular disease, JACC 43 (2004) 179–18449.
[17] M. Bocchio, et al., Endothelial cell activation in men with erectile dysfunction without cardiovascular risk factors and overt vascular damage, J. Urol. 171 (2004) 1601–1604.
[18] P. Montorsi, et al., Association between erectile dysfunction and coronary artery disease. Role of coronary clinical presentation and extent of coronary vessel involvement: the COBRA trial, Eur. Heart J. 27 (22) (2006) 2632–2649.
[19] S. Jacobsen, et al., Erectile dysfunction and acute myocardial infarction: the Olmsted county study, Circulation 108 (Supplement IV) (2003) IV–752.
[20] W.A. Blumentals, A. Gomez-Caminero, S.J. Vannappagari, Should erectile dysfunction be considered as a marker for acute myocardial infarction? Results from a retrospective cohort study, Int. J. Impot. Res. 16 (2004) 350–353.
[21] P. Stroberg, E. Frick, H. Hedelin, Is erectile dysfunction really a clinically useful predictor of cardiovascular disease? Scand. J. Urol. Nephrol. 39 (2005) 62–65.
[22] I.M. Thompson, et al., Erectile dysfunction and subsequent cardiovascular disease, JAMA 294 (2005) 2996–3002.
[23] R.B. D'Agostino, et al., Validation of the Framingham heart disease prediction score: results of a multiple ethnic groups investigation, JAMA 286 (2001) 180–187.
[24] R.M. Conroy, et al., Estimation of ten-year risk of fatal cardiovascular disease in Europe: the SCORE project, Eur. Heart J. 24 (2003) 987–1003.
[25] J.B. Kostis, et al., Sexual dysfunction and cardiac risk (the Second Princeton Consensus Conference), Am. J. Cardiol. 96 (2005) 313–321.
[26] P. Greenland, S.C. Smith, S.M. Grundy, Improving coronary heart disease risk assessment in asymptomatic people, Circulation 104 (2001) 1863–1867.
[27] Executive summary of the third report of the national cholesterol education program (NCEP) expert panel on detection, evaluation, and treatment of high blood cholesterol in adults (Adult treatment panel III), JAMA 285 (2001) 2486–2497.
[28] P. Montorsi, et al., Association between erectile dysfunction and coronary artery disease: matching the right target with the right test in the right patient, Eur. Urol. 50 (2006) 721–731.

ELSEVIER

International Congress Series 1303 (2007) 65–69

www.ics-elsevier.com

Cerebrovascular disease in type 2 diabetes

Markku Laakso *, Johanna Kuusisto

Department of Medicine, University of Kuopio, Kuopio, 70210 Finland

Abstract. Type 2 diabetes is associated with at least 2-fold elevated risk for all macrovascular complications, coronary heart disease, stroke and peripheral vascular disease. The prevalence and incidence of hemorrhagic stroke is not higher among subjects with type 2 diabetes than in non-diabetic subjects. Therefore, an excess risk of stroke is due to high occurrence of ischemic strokes. High LDL cholesterol, elevated blood pressure, smoking, low HDL cholesterol, high levels of total triglycerides and insulin, central obesity, impaired glucose tolerance and atrial fibrillation have been associated with the risk of stroke. Diabetic patients with stroke should receive effective antihypertensive therapy, lipid-lowering medication, medication to obtain good glycemic control, and anti-platelet therapy. Surgical revascularization is indicated in patients with hemodynamically significant internal carotid artery atherosclerosis independently of symptoms. Patients with atrial fibrillation should be on anticoagulation therapy. © 2007 Published by Elsevier B.V.

Keywords: Type 2 diabetes; Cerebrovascular disease; Hyperglycaemia

1. Introduction

Diabetes mellitus affects about 3–5% of western populations. The prevalence of this disorder is rapidly increasing almost in all countries, and diabetes will be one of the main threats to human health in the 21st century. Changes in the human environment and in human behavior and lifestyle, in conjunction with genetic susceptibility, have resulted in a dramatic increase in the incidence and prevalence of diabetes in the world. Most of this increase is due to an epidemic of type 2 diabetes (T2DM) because this subtype accounts for 90% of cases globally.

Chronic hyperglycemia is associated with long-term complications, especially in the eyes, kidneys, nerves, heart, and blood vessels. More than half of patients with T2DM die

* Corresponding author. Tel.: +358 17 172151; fax: +358 17 173993.
E-mail address: markku.laakso@kuh.fi (M. Laakso).

0531-5131/ © 2007 Published by Elsevier B.V.
doi:10.1016/j.ics.2007.03.017

of cardiovascular diseases (CVD), especially of coronary heart disease (CHD) and stroke. Therefore, the 'epidemic' of T2DM will be followed by the 'epidemic' of diabetes-related CVD.

T2DM is preceded by a long period of asymptomatic hyperglycemia, associated with the clustering or cardiovascular risk factors. In this pre-diabetic state, postprandial or postglucose levels are mildly elevated, whereas fasting blood glucose can usually be maintained within the near-normal range. Very often these risk individuals also have the metabolic syndrome [1], a clustering of other cardiovascular risk factors, e.g. abdominal obesity, elevated levels of total triglycerides, low levels of high-density lipoprotein (HDL) cholesterol and elevated blood pressure. These individuals are at a high risk or developing CVD, including stroke.

Type 2 diabetes is associated with at least 2-fold elevated risk for all macrovascular complications, coronary heart disease (CHD), stroke and peripheral vascular disease. Classical risk factors, high low-density lipoprotein (LDL) cholesterol, elevated blood pressure, and smoking, increase the risk of CVD similarly to non-diabetic subjects [2]. However, the absolute risk for CVD is substantially higher among patients with T2DM.

2. Clinical characteristics of stroke among patients with type 2 diabetes

Barker et al. [3] reported that beyond the fourth decade of life the frequency and severity of cerebral atherosclerosis was doubled in diabetic subjects compared to non-diabetic individuals. Grunnet et al. [4] found that in subjects aged from 30 to 70 years nearly twice as many diabetic subjects as non-diabetic subjects had moderate or severe cerebral atherosclerosis, whereas above 70 years of age this difference became less striking. Patients with type 2 diabetes have more extracranial atherosclerosis. Several clinical series of diabetic patients and population-based studies have shown that diabetic patients have about 2-fold higher risk for stroke compared to control subjects [2].

Stroke has special characteristics in patients with T2DM compared to non-diabetic subjects presented in Table 1 (modified from [5]). The prevalence and incidence of hemorrhagic stroke is not higher among subjects with T2DM than in non-diabetic subjects. Therefore, an excess risk of stroke is due to high occurrence of ischemic strokes. In patients with T2DM the ratio of ischemic stroke/hemorrhagic stroke is 10:1, whereas in non-diabetic subjects it is 5:1. Furthermore, the relative risk for stroke in patients with T2DM is especially high in subjects <55 years [6] and in women. Diabetes doubles the risk of

Table 1
Clinical characteristics of stroke in patients with type 2 diabetes

Ratio of ischemic stroke vs. hemorrhagic stroke, 10:1
10-fold higher stroke risk than in non-diabetic subjects, if age <55 years
Risk for women higher than for men
Infratentorial infarcts more common than in non-diabetic subjects
Lacunar infarcts more common than in non-diabetic subjects
Infarcts located in brainstem, cerebellar or midbrain region more common than in non-diabetic subjects
Infarction size not different from that in non-diabetic individuals

recurrence of stroke [7], and increases total and stroke-related mortality [8]. Localization of stroke is also different between diabetic and non-diabetic subjects. Intratentoral and lacunar infarcts are more common in patients with T2DM than in non-diabetic individuals, as well as stroke-related dementia [9]. The size of infarct in stroke patients is not different between diabetic and non-diabetic subjects.

3. Risk factors for stroke

In addition to classic risk factors, high LDL cholesterol, elevated blood pressure and smoking, low HDL cholesterol, high levels of triglycerides and insulin, central obesity, impaired glucose tolerance and atrial fibrillation have been associated with the risk of stroke [10,11]. Thus, insulin resistance must be a central component in the risk of stroke. In fact, insulin resistance syndrome has been shown to predict stroke in population-based studies [12].

In insulin-resistant states skeletal muscle glucose uptake is impaired, leading to high insulin levels in circulating blood since the pancreas compensates for impaired insulin action by secreting more insulin. Glucose and free fatty acid (FFA) levels are elevated which increases the risk of atherothrombosis. Insulin resistance in adipose tissue leads to increased lipolysis and high FFA flux into the liver where it stimulates the production of very low density lipoprotein (VLDL) particles, and thus dyslipidemia (high triglycerides, low HDL cholesterol, small and dense LDL particles) [1]. Furthermore, adipose tissue secretes important adipocytokines, for example tumor necrosis factor-α, interleukin-6 and adiponectin. In people with high amount of visceral fat, the levels of cytokines, adhesion molecules, and inflammatory markers are elevated whereas adiponectin concentration is low [13]. All these changes contribute to accelerated atherothrombosis. In response to cytokines the liver produces C-reactive protein, plasminogen activator inhibitor 1 and fibrinogen which lead to enhanced thrombus formation and impaired fibrinolysis. Finally, in insulin resistant states endothelial dysfunction is present, since nitric oxide production is not stimulated.

In T2DM the degree of hyperglycemia and long duration of diabetes are risk factors for stroke [14]. Hyperglycemia has several deleterious effects on the risk of atherothrombosis. Glucose toxicity further impairs insulin signaling, glucose metabolism and endothelial function. Furthermore, hyperglycemia stimulates the MAP kinase pathway leading to elevated synthesis of adhesion molecules and endothelin 1, as well as to the stimulation of vascular smooth muscle cell proliferation, and changes in the arterial wall. Hyperglycemia also leads to the formation of advanced glycation end products, increased oxidative stress, and abnormalities in other cardiovascular risk factors [15]. Finally, in diabetes there are abnormalities in platelet function and coagulation. These abnormalities increase intrinsic platelet activation and decrease endogenous inhibitors of platelet activity, and augment blood coagulation [16].

Although several potential risk factors for accelerated atherothrombosis have been identified, it is possible to measure only a few of them in clinical practice. UK Prospective Diabetes Study (UKPDS) evaluated risk factors for stroke case fatality (Table 2). This study demonstrated that from modifiable risk factors particularly elevated blood pressure and hemoglobin A1c were strong predictors for fatal stroke [17]. Our study has shown that in addition to risk factors found

Table 2
Risk factors predicting stroke case fatality in the UK Prospective Diabetes Study in multivariate model [17]

Risk factor	Odds ratio and their 95% confidence intervals	*p* value
Gender (women vs. men)	2.33 (1.11–4.91)	0.0253
Hemoglobin A1c (per 1%)	1.37 (1.09–1.72)	0.0071
Systolic blood pressure (per 10 mm Hg)	1.29 (1.04–1.54)	0.0040
Subsequent stroke vs. first stroke	12.6(4.34–36.7)	<0.0001
White cell count (per 10^{-9} l)	0.82 (0.67–0.97)	0.0218

in the UKPDS, dyslipidemia (low HDL cholesterol, and high triglycerides) [18] and proteinuria [19] are strong risk factors for stroke in type 2 diabetic patients.

4. Prevention of stroke

Diabetic patients with stroke should receive effective antihypertensive therapy, lipid-lowering medication, medication to obtain good glycemic control, and anti-platelet therapy. Surgical revascularization is indicated in patients with hemodynamically significant internal carotid artery atherosclerosis independently of symptoms [15]. Patients with atrial fibrillation should be on anticoagulation therapy.

Intervention trials have provided support for rigorous blood pressure control in the prevention of stroke in diabetic patients. In the UKPDS tight blood pressure with atenolol or captopril resulted in 44% relative risk reduction in fatal and nonfatal stroke compared with the control group [20]. Also treatment with calcium channels blockers, diuretics, other ACE inhibitors and angiotensin receptor blockers has been shown to prevent stroke events [21]. Blood pressure reduction *per se* rather than the choice of a specific agent is of primary importance.

A prospective meta-analysis of data from 90 056 individuals of 14 randomized statin trials has been recently published [22]. The relative risk reduction of ischemic stroke by statin treatment was 19% (95% confidence interval (CI) 11–26%), but no effect on hemorrhagic stroke was found. The relative risk reduction was of similar magnitude in non-diabetic and diabetic subjects.

Meta-analysis of 6 trials on the effect of glucose lowering in type 2 diabetic patients included 4472 patients and 303 cerebrovascular events [23]. This meta-analysis showed that the relative risk of stroke was reduced by 42% (95% CI 26–54%) by intensive glucose control. The first study aiming to investigate the effect of improving insulin sensitivity on cardiovascular disease was the PROactive Study (PROspective pioglitAzone Clinical Trial In macroVascular Events) [24]. This trial randomized 5238 patients with T2DM, who had evidence of macrovascular disease, to receive pioglitazone 45 mg or matching placebo. The primary endpoint of all-cause mortality, non-fatal myocardial infarction, stroke, acute coronary syndrome, endovascular or surgical intervention in the coronary or leg arteries, and amputation above the ankle was not significantly reduced (hazard ratio 0.90, 95% CI 0.80–1.02, $p=0.095$). However, the number of subjects with stroke was considerably less in the pioglitazone group than in the placebo group (76 vs. 96).

Aspirin therapy reduces the risk of stroke in adults who are at increased risk for cardiovascular disease. Therefore, all patients with T2DM should be on aspirin therapy, if contraindications are not present [25]. A dose of 100 mg is recommended, but diabetic patients may need a larger dose. Patients with atrial fibrillation benefit from anticoagulation. Finally, diabetic patients with hemodynamically significant internal carotid artery atherosclerosis benefit from surgical revascularization.

References

[1] M. Laakso, Insulin resistance and coronary heart disease, Curr. Opin. Lipidol. 7 (1996) 217–226.

[2] K. Pyörälä, M. Laakso, M. Uusitupa, Diabetes and atherosclerosis: an epidemiologic view, Diabetes/Metabolism Rev. 3 (1987) 463–524.

[3] A.B. Baker, J. Kinnard, A. Iannone, Cerebrovascular disease: VIII. Role of nutritional factors, Neurology 13 (1963) 486–491.

[4] M.L. Grunnet, Cerebrovascular: diabetes and cerebral atherosclerosis, Neurology 13 (1963) 486–491.

[5] I. Idris, G.A. Thompson, J.C. Sharma, Diabetes mellitus and stroke, Int. J. Clin. Pract. 60 (2006) 48–56.

[6] R.X. You, et al., Risk factors for stroke due to cerebral infarction in young adults, Stroke 28 (1997) 1913–1918.

[7] G.J. Hankey, et al., Long-term risk of first recurrent stroke in the Perth Community Stroke Study, Stroke 29 (1998) 2491–5000.

[8] J. Tuomilehto, et al., Diabetes mellitus as a risk factor for death from stroke, Stroke 27 (1996) 210–215.

[9] J.A. Luchsinger, et al., Diabetes mellitus and risk of Alzheimer's disease and dementia with stroke in a multiethnic cohort, Am. J. Epidemiol. 154 (2001) 635–641.

[10] A.R. Folsom, et al., Prospective associations of fasting insulin, body fat distribution, and diabetes with risk of ischemic stroke, Diabetes Care 22 (1999) 1077–1083.

[11] R.L. Sacco, et al., High-density lipoprotein cholesterol and ischemic stroke in patients with diagnosed with TIA, Neurology 28 (2001) 280–285.

[12] M. Pyörälä, et al., Insulin resistance syndrome predicts the risk of coronary heart disease and stroke in healthy middle-aged men: the 22-year follow-up results of the Helsinki Policemen Study, Arterioscler. Thromb. Vasc. Biol. 20 (2000) 538–544.

[13] U. Salmenniemi, et al., Multiple abnormalities in glucose and energy metabolism, and coordinated changes in levels of adiponectin, cytokines and adhesion molecules in subjects with the metabolic syndrome, Circulation 110 (2004) 3842–3848.

[14] J. Kuusisto, et al., Non-insulin-dependent diabetes and its metabolic control are important predictors of stroke in elderly subjects, Stroke 25 (1994) 1157–1564.

[15] J.A. Beckman, M.A. Creager, Diabetes and atherosclerosis. Epidemiology, pathophysiology, and management, JAMA 287 (2002) 2570–2581.

[16] A.I. Vinik, et al., Platelet dysfunction in type 2 diabetes, Diabetes Care 24 (2001) 1476–1485.

[17] R.J. Stevens, et al., Risk factors for myocardial infarction case fatality and stroke case fatality in type 2 diabetes. UKPDS 66, Diabetes Care 27 (2004) 201–207.

[18] S. Lehto, et al., Predictors of stroke in middle-aged patients with non-insulin-dependent diabetes, Stroke 27 (1996) 63–68.

[19] H. Miettinen, et al., Proteinuria predicts stroke and other atherosclerotic vascular disease events in nondiabetic and non-insulin-dependent diabetic subjects, Stroke 27 (1996) 2033–2039.

[20] T.M. Davis, et al., Risk factors for stroke in type 2 diabetes mellitus. United Kingdom Prospective Diabetes Study (UKPDS) 29, Arch. Intern. Med. 159 (1999) 1097–1103.

[21] J.R. Sowers, Treatment of hypertension in patients with diabetes, Arch. Intern. Med. 164 (2004) 1850–1857.

[22] Cholesterol Treatment Trialist' (CTT) Collaborators, Efficacy and safety of cholesterol-lowering treatment: prospective meta-analysis of data from 90 056 participants in 14 randomised trials of statins, Lancet 366 (2005) 1267–1278.

[23] C. Stettler, et al., Glycemic control and macrovascular disease in type 1 and 2 diabetes mellitus: meta-analysis of randomized trials, Am. Heart. J. 152 (2006) 27–38.

[24] J.A. Dormandy, et al., Secondary prevention of macrovascular events in patients with type 2 diabetes in the PROactive Study (PROspective pioglitAzone Clinical Trial In macroVascular Events): a randomised controlled trial, Lancet 366 (2005) 1279–1289.

[25] JA. Coldwell, Aspirin therapy in diabetes, Diabetes Care (2004) S72–S73 27 (Suppl).

International Congress Series 1303 (2007) 70–73

www.ics-elsevier.com

Coronary heart disease in diabetes

Angelo Avogaro*, Gianpaolo Fadini,
Saula Vigili de Kreutzenberg, Antonio Tiengo

Department of Clinical and Experimental Medicine, University of Padova, Italy

Abstract. Type Diabetes Mellitus is a chronic disease, whose incidence is alarmingly growing. It is associated with severe metabolic abnormalities and increased cardiovascular morbidity and mortality. The first detectable alteration in the pathogenesis of atherosclerosis is endothelial dysfunction which is linked to alteration in microcirculation. Detection of microvascular dysfunction in diabetes would force physician to implement early aggressive therapeutic intervention. © 2007 Published by Elsevier B.V.

Keywords: Coronary heart disease; Diabetes; Endothelial dysfunction; Oxidative stress; Myocardial perfusion

1. Introduction

Macrovascular disease is the main cause of death in type 1 and type 2 diabetes. Microvascular complications are also important contributory factors of macrovascular disease. The EPIC–Norfolk (European Prospective Investigation into Cancer in Norfolk) study showed a correlation between coronary heart disease (CHD) risk, and increasing HbA1c as well as all-cause mortality and increasing HbA1c: each increase in HbA1c of 1% was associated with a 20–30% increase in mortality from a CV event [1]. Thus the relationship between diabetes and CHD is not a threshold but a continuous one. Most risks are determined possibly not only to dysglycaemia itself but rather to coexisting risk factors such as hyperlipidemia, hypertension, and pro-inflammatory state.

* Corresponding author. Department of Clinical and Experimental Medicine, Policlinico Universitario, Via Giustiniani 2, 35128, Padova, Italy. Tel.: +39 0498212178; fax: +39 0498754179.
E-mail address: angelo.avogaro@unipd.it (A. Avogaro).

0531-5131/ © 2007 Published by Elsevier B.V.
doi:10.1016/j.ics.2007.04.006

2. Micro and macrovascular disease

The prevailing concept is that CHD is mostly present in type 2 rather than in type 1 diabetic patients: this belief has been confuted by several studies showing that the burden of CHD is similar in both conditions [2]. About half of the patients with diabetes develop microalbuminuria at some point. Approximately one third will progress to proteinuria, one third will remain microalbuminuric. There is an increasing evidence that micro- and macrovascular complications of diabetes share certain pathophysiological mechanisms. This may explain why microangiopathy has been associated with macroangiopathy and with mortality. In type 2 diabetic patients, increasing excretion of microalbuminuria progressively enhances the relative risk of myocardial infarction, and CV death [3]. Similar observation has been performed also in type 1 diabetic patients: subjects with diabetic nephropathy have a significantly higher incidence of CHD than those without [4]. The presence of diabetic retinopathy also identifies patients at risk for CHD. The EURODIAB Prospective Complications Study has shown that type 1 diabetic patients with nonproliferative or proliferative retinopathy have an increased risk for all-cause mortality and incident CVD [5]. The presence of cardiovascular risk factors explained the associations to a large extent, except for the associations with proliferative retinopathy, which suggests that other shared mechanisms may be involved. High blood glucose is an extremely detrimental factor for the retinal microvasculature. The hyperglycaemic damage to the retinal vessels results in increased permeability, endothelial detachment and pericyte loss. Consequences are blood and serum leakage from the intravascular to the extravascular space and progressive decline in retinal blood flow. Retinal ischemia and release of angiogenic factors stimulate the proliferation of microvessels ultimately leading to proliferative retinopathy. Recently, intriguing novelties have added to this classic pathogenetic model of diabetic retinopathy. It has been shown in animals that bone marrow-derived cells are mobilized and recruited at sites of retinal neovascularization in response to VEGF and SDF-1 [6]. Therefore, not only local endothelial cells, but also the so called endothelial progenitor cells (EPCs) may be involved in the development of proliferative retinopathy. We have studied in vivo the levels of CD34+ and CD34+ KDR+ EPCs and in vitro differentiation of EPCs in type 2 diabetic patients with various combinations of PAD and DR [7]. While levels of CD34+ KDR+ cells and endothelial differentiation of cultured progenitors were selectively reduced in PAD patients, generic CD34+ progenitors were reduced in DR patients, which showed instead higher clonogenic potential and enhanced endothelial differentiation of cultured EPCs.

3. Microcirculation in the heart

Several years ago Factor and colleagues demonstrated considerable microvascular abnormalities within the heart of hypertensive-diabetic rats [8]. Thus the natural history of CHD in the diabetic heart starts early in the course of the disease not only as a disease specific of the epicardial vessels but as a small vessel disease. There is an extensive evidence of an independent and cumulative effect of postprandial hyperglycemia on endothelial dysfunction and oxidative stress generation; that regional myocardial blood flow redistribution is a cause of postprandial angina pectoris; that reduced availability of nitric oxide during hyperglycemia. We have clearly shown that acute hyperglycemia in the postprandial state is associated with myocardial perfusion defects in type 2 diabetic patients [9]. These defects are secondary to deterioration in microvascular function, which may represent an early marker of the atherogenic process in the coronary circulation. From a clinical point of view, controlling postprandial hyperglycemia and myocardial perfusion defects may constitute important goals in the treatment of the disease. Our data indirectly support the observation of the DIAD (Detection of Silent Myocardial Ischemia in Asymptomatic Diabetics) study which has highlighted the scale of the problem of CHD and silent ischemia in a population of asymptomatic diabetic patients [10]. In a middle-aged or elderly patient population (mean age 61 years) with high proportions of patients with dyslipidemia (58%), hypertension (65%), a history of smoking (58%), or at least 2 cardiovascular risk factors (60%), adenosine electrocardiography (ECG)-gated technetium-99 m sestamibi single-photon emission computed tomography (SPECT) showed that myocardial perfusion alterations were detectable in 22% of patients. Perfusion abnormalities were reversible in 88% of these patients (indicating ischemia), although 4% demonstrated irreversible abnormalities (indicating scar tissue) and 8% demonstrated both reversible and irreversible perfusion defects. Cardiac neuropathy was an independent predictor of abnormal myocardial perfusion. The results of the DIAD study are consistent with other studies in diabetic patients who were asymptomatic, in which the prevalence of abnormal perfusion scans ranged from 21% to 59% [11]. In conclusion we can assert that 1. microvascular complications are important determinant of macrovascular disease; 2. early alterations in coronary microcirculation are detectable without atherosclerotic burden in epicardial coronary vessels, especially during the postprandial period; 3. a large proportion of patients has markedly abnormal (moderate-to-large) myocardial perfusion abnormalities.

4. The need of an early identification of CHD in diabetic patients

The Consensus Development Conference on the diagnosis of CAD in people with diabetes of the American Diabetes Association (ADA) recommends performing stress screening for CHD in asymptomatic patients with two or more additional risk factors [12]. It was stated that asymptomatic diabetic patients with ≥ 1 RF do not require cardiac testing. However, we have shown that an "aggressive" diagnostic approach, requiring coronary angiography in asymptomatic DM2 patients with ≤ 1 associated risk factor for CHD and abnormal myocardial perfusion, identified patients with a subclinical CAD characterized by a more favourable angiographic anatomy [13]. Moreover, the criterion of ≤ 2 risk factors did not help to identify asymptomatic patients with a higher prevalence of CAD and is only related to a more severe CAD with unfavourable coronary anatomy. For these reasons current guidelines and reports from European and US expert societies in cardiovascular medicine recognize the potential utility of myocardial perfusion in risk stratification of diabetic patients but do not widely recommend its use in patients without symptoms of CHD. Of note, patients with an abnormal ECG indicating previous infarction or ischemia should be referred for stress testing according to the Guidelines of the American Diabetes Association. Indeed, it was recently demonstrated that the presence of Q waves on the ECG was highly predictive not only of severely abnormal myocardial perfusion but of extensive CHD burden [14].

5. Conclusions

In diabetic patients, CHD should be prevented by keeping glycated haemoglobin as low as possible aiming for <6.5%. Blood pressure should be as low as possible aiming for <130/80 mm Hg or <125/75 mm Hg if proteinuria is present, if the glomerular filtration is <60 ml/min/1.73 m^2, or if the patient has cardiovascular disease. Statins should be prescribed for patients over 40 or under 40 if microvascular or macrovascular complications, hypertension, metabolic syndrome, or a family history of cardiovascular disease is present. Low density lipoprotein–cholesterol should be <70 mg/dl. Aspirin should be prescribed for all patients over 40; smoking should be banned and patients encouraged to maintain an ideal body weight. However aggressive diagnostic approach must be implemented so that both CHD and the so called diabetic cardiomyopathy should be detected in a subclinical phase. Not only an ECG but also a myocardial perfusion study should be obtained along with an extensive screening for the presence of microvascular complications.

References

[1] K.T. Khaw, et al., Association of hemoglobin A1c with cardiovascular disease and mortality in adults: the European prospective investigation into cancer in Norfolk, Ann. Intern. Med. 141 (6) (2004) 413–420.

[2] P. Valsania, et al., Severity of coronary artery disease in young patients with insulin-dependent diabetes mellitus, Am. Heart J. 122 (3 Pt 1) (1991) 695–700.

[3] H. Gerstein, et al., HOPE Study Investigators. Albuminuria and risk of cardiovascular events, death, and heart failure in diabetic and nondiabetic individuals, JAMA 286 (4) (2001) 421–426.

[4] J. Tuomilehto, et al., Incidence of cardiovascular disease in Type 1 (insulin-dependent) diabetic subjects with and without diabetic nephropathy in Finland, Diabetologia 41 (7) (1998) 784–790.

[5] M.V. van Hecke, et al., EURODIAB prospective complications study Diabetic retinopathy is associated with mortality and cardiovascular disease incidence: the EURODIAB prospective complications study, Diabetes Care 28 (6) (2005) 1383–1389.

[6] K.G. Csaky, et al., Recruitment of marrow-derived endothelial cells to experimental choroidal neovascularization by local expression of vascular endothelial growth factor, Exp. Eye Res. 78 (2004) 1107–1116.

[7] G.P. Fadini, et al., Endothelial progenitor cells and the diabetic paradox, Diabetes Care 29 (3) (2006) 714–716.

[8] S.M. Factor, et al., Coronary microvascular abnormalities in the hypertensive-diabetic rat. A primary cause of cardiomyopathy? Am. J. Pathol. 116 (1) (1984) 9–20.

[9] R. Scognamiglio, C. Negut, S.V. De Kreutzenberg, A. Tiengo, A. Avogaro, Postprandial myocardial perfusion in healthy subjects and in type 2 diabetic patients, Circulation 112 (2) (2005 Jul 12) 179–184 (Electronic publication 2005 Jul 5).

[10] F.J. Wackers, et al., The Detection of Silent Myocardial Ischemia in Asymptomatic Diabetics (DIAD) study, Diabetes Care 27 (2004) 1954–1961.

[11] J.J. Bax, R.O. Bonow, D. Tschope, S.E. Inzucchi, E. Barrett, Global Dialogue Group for the Evaluation of Cardiovascular Risk in Patients With Diabetes. The potential of myocardial perfusion scintigraphy for risk stratification of asymptomatic patients with type 2 diabetes, J. Am. Coll. Cardiol. 48 (4) (2006 Aug 15) 754–760 (Electronic publication 2006 Jul 24).

[12] E.J. Barett, et al., Consensus development conference on the diagnosis of coronary heart disease in people with diabetes, Diabetes Care 21 (1998) 1551–1559.

[13] R. Scognamiglio, C. Negut, A. Ramondo, A. Tiengo, A. Avogaro, Detection of coronary artery disease in asymptomatic patients with type 2 diabetes mellitus, J. Am. Coll. Cardiol. 47 (1) (2006 Jan 3) 65–71 (Electronic publication 2005 Dec 9).

[14] N. Rajagopalan, et al., Identifying high-risk asymptomatic diabetic patients who are candidates for screening stress single-photon emission computed tomography imaging, J Am Coll Cardiol 45 (2005) 43–49.

International Congress Series 1303 (2007) 74–82

ELSEVIER

www.ics-elsevier.com

Atherothrombotic disease and the metabolic syndrome

Giovanni Daví *, Francesca Santilli

Center of Excellence on Aging, "G. d'Annunzio" University Foundation, Via Colle dell'Ara, 66013 Chieti, Italy

Abstract. The metabolic syndrome (MS) is a disorder characterized by a higher risk of cardiovascular disease (CVD) and by a clustering of cardiovascular risk factors, which *per se* do not sufficiently explain the excess vascular risk attributed to this syndrome. The *core* abnormality accounting for most of the features of the MS consists in the resistance to the metabolic and vascular actions of insulin, leading to chronic proinflammatory state, increased oxidative stress, procoagulant/anti-fibrinolytic state, coupled with platelet hyperaggregability.

We have previously provided evidence of persistent thromboxane (TXA_2)-dependent platelet activation in association with features of the MS, including visceral obesity and diabetes. We suggested a cause-and-effect relationship between oxidative stress and platelet activation by showing the linear relationship between the excretion rates of 8-*iso*-prostaglandin (PG)$F_{2\alpha}$ and 11-dehydro-TXB_2, markers of in vivo lipid peroxidation and platelet activation, respectively, and their downregulation following improvement of glycemic control in diabetes mellitus or weight loss in obesity. Subsequent observations elucidated the concept that insulin resistance *per se* is a major determinant of increased platelet activation in obesity, independently of underlying inflammation.

Interventions such as caloric restriction, exercise and insulin sensitizing agents may favourably modulate most of the metabolic abnormalities predisposing to atherothrombosis in the MS. © 2007 Elsevier B.V. All rights reserved.

Keywords: Metabolic syndrome; Atherothrombosis; Oxidative stress; Inflammation; Platelet activation

1. Introduction

The metabolic syndrome (MS) is a disorder associated with accelerated atherosclerosis and characterized by a clustering of cardiovascular risk factors [1]. The age-adjusted prevalence of

* Corresponding author. Tel.: +39 0871 541312; fax: +39 0871 541261.
E-mail address: gdavi@unich.it (G. Daví).

doi:10.1016/j.ics.2007.03.023

the syndrome is 23% in the US population aged more than 20 years [2]. In the Framingham Study, MS alone predicts about 25% of new cardiovascular disease (CVD) cases [3]. The ATP III report identified six components of the MS that may predispose to CVD: abdominal obesity; atherogenic dyslipidemia; raised blood pressure; insulin resistance and/or glucose intolerance; proinflammatory state, recognized clinically by elevations of C-reactive protein (CRP), and prothrombotic state characterized by increased plasma plasminogen activator inhibitor (PAI)-1 and fibrinogen. Mutual interactions between these factors reinforced by several positive loops largely account for the pathogenesis of the MS [4] and contribute to the development of atherothrombosis in this setting.

However, the known metabolic risk factors associated with this syndrome do not sufficiently explain the excess vascular risk attributed to this syndrome.

2. Determinants of atherothrombosis in the metabolic syndrome

2.1. Obesity and insulin resistance

2.1.1. Low-grade inflammation coupled with oxidative stress

Over the past decade, obesity has been associated with inflammation by demonstrating that tumor necrosis factor-α is constitutively expressed by adipose tissue. Obese adipose tissue is characterized by inflammation and progressive infiltration by macrophages as obesity develops [5]. A low-grade chronic inflammatory state, characterized by increased levels of inflammatory proteins and acute-phase proteins, is present in patients with obesity and MS. In a large cohort of women participating to the Women's Health Study, a strong linear increase was detected in CRP levels as the number of component of the MS increased. In addition, baseline CRP levels add clinically relevant prognostic information concerning future vascular risk [6]. Furthermore, CRP has been shown to increase PAI-1 expression and activity in human aortic endothelial cells [7].

Adipose tissue, far from being an inert organ, has the capacity to secrete biologically active mediators [8]. They may influence cardiovascular risk through their involvement not only in body weight homeostasis, but also in inflammation, coagulation, fibrinolysis, endothelial dysfunction, insulin resistance and atherosclerosis [9].

Adiponectin, an adipokine with proved anti-atherogenic and anti-inflammatory properties, which is inversely related to insulin resistance, has been recently shown to act as an endogenous antithrombotic factor, since its overexpression attenuated thrombus formation in mice [10]. Moreover, circulating adiponectin is reduced and independently related to reduced IL-10 levels in android obese women [11]. In addition, the increase of circulating leptin, in obese women, is associated with markers of hemostatic system [12].

Activation of intracellular pathways by several mediators promotes the development of insulin resistance. Increasing adiposity activates either JNK and IKKβ [13], both through receptor and nonreceptor pathways. Proinflammatory cytokines such as TNFα and IL-1β activate JNK and IKKβ/NF-κB through classical receptor-mediated mechanisms. JNK and IKKβ/NF-κB are also activated by pattern recognition receptors (surface proteins that recognize foreign substances), including toll-like receptors and receptors for advanced glycosylation end-products (RAGE) [14]. In addition to proinflammatory cytokine and pattern recognition receptors, cellular stresses activate reactive oxygen species, through mechanisms possibly involving activation of NADPH oxidase [15]. It has been suggested that obesity *per se* may induce systemic oxidative stress in accumulated fat via NADPH oxidase activation, that is, at least in part, the underlying cause of dysregulation of adipocitokines and development of MS [15]. Recently, NADPH oxidase activation has been proposed as a potential target mechanism for MS [16].

The proinflammatory state of obesity and metabolic syndrome originates with excessive caloric intake and is probably a result of overnutrition. The proinflammatory state coupled with oxidative stress induces insulin resistance which promotes inflammation further through an increase in free fatty acids (FFA) concentration and interference with the anti-inflammatory effect of insulin; moreover, FFA release from adipocytes induces endothelial dysfunction due to increased reactive oxygen species (ROS) generation and oxidative stress [17].

The *core* abnormality which may account for most of the features predisposing to atherothrombosis in MS consists in insulin resistance. It is characterized by pathway-specific impairment in phosphatidylinositol 3-kinase-dependent signaling, which overdrives unaffected MAP-kinase-dependent pathways, leading to an imbalance between production of NO and secretion of endothelin-1, and increased growth and mitogenesis in vascular endothelium [18]. Thus, insulin resistance couples vascular and metabolic pathophysiology by triggering a series of mechanisms, including inflammation, endothelial dysfunction and vasoconstriction, predisposing insulin resistant individuals to accelerated atherosclerosis and thrombosis [19].

2.1.2. Functional read-outs of enhanced inflammation and oxidative stress: coagulative and platelet activation

Patients with MS have enhanced plasma levels of the inflammatory and prothrombotic molecule CD40 ligand (CD40L), and of prothrombin fragment 1+2 (F1+2), with a significant correlation between the two biochemical variables [20]. CD40L is derived from platelets by more than 95%, stored in the cytoplasm of unstimulated platelets and expressed on the surface of platelets within seconds of platelet activation and then cleaved to generate a soluble, trimeric fragment, sCD40L. It may be involved in a self-perpetuating feedback loop, whereby it binds platelet-bound CD40 leading to further proteolysis of membrane bound CD40L, with consequent generation of further sCD40L [21]. CD40/CD40L interaction occurs on virtually all of the cells involved in the processes of atherosclerosis at all stages, such as vascular endothelial cells, macrophages, activated T lymphocytes, and platelets, triggering a series of events occurring in the vascular wall and in the circulation during the ongoing inflammatory response.

Resistance to the metabolic and vascular actions of insulin [22] leads to a chronic proinflammatory state, an increased oxidative stress with augmented ROS generation, a procoagulant/anti-fibrinolytic state, coupled with platelet hyperaggregability. In this regard, we demonstrated a significant association between insulin resistance and markers of inflammation and thrombin generation. Indeed, obese women with impaired insulin sensitivity had significantly higher levels of CRP, TGF-β, PAI-1, FVIIa and F1+2, compared to either healthy controls or non insulin resistant obese women [23]. Moreover, insulin resistance elicits the gene transcription of PAI-1, which exerts anti-fibrinolytic actions, thus promoting a procoagulant state in the metabolic syndrome [24]. PAI-1 levels are significantly higher in android obese women compared with gynoid obese or non-obese women. A direct correlation exists between PAI-1 levels and oxidative stress, as assessed by 8-*iso*-prostaglandin (PG)$F_{2\alpha}$ urinary excretion, in obese women [25].

In vitro and *in vivo* studies have demonstrated that in obese individuals and in obese type 2 diabetics the antiaggregating effect of insulin is blunted, consistent with the finding that human platelets, which have insulin receptors that modulate platelet function, are sites of insulin resistance [22].

In this regard, we have previously provided evidence of persistent thromboxane-dependent platelet activation in association with features of the metabolic syndrome, including visceral obesity [26]. In this setting we characterized a putative biochemical link between obesity and platelet activation, by investigating in vivo formation of F_2-isoprostanes, as reflected by urinary excretion of 8-*iso*-$PGF_{2\alpha}$, in vivo marker of oxidative stress. We observed that obese women, in particular those with visceral obesity, had higher levels of lipid peroxidation, as assessed by urinary 8-*iso*-$PGF_{2\alpha}$, and platelet activation, as reflected by urinary excretion of the TXA_2 enzymatic metabolite 11-dehydro-TXB_2, when compared to age-matched non-obese women. When plasma CRP concentrations were divided in quartiles, the excretion rates of 8-*iso*-$PGF_{2\alpha}$ and 11-dehydro-TXB_2 significantly increased from the first to the fourth quartiles. On multiple regression analysis, plasma levels of CRP and the waist-to-hip-ratio predicted the rate of isoprostane formation. We also examined the short term effects of a weight loss program by assessing in android obese women changes associated with caloric restriction. Successful weight loss was associated with a statistically significant reduction in both urinary metabolites.

The cause-and-effect relationship between oxidative stress and platelet activation is demonstrated by the linear relationship between the excretion rates of 8-*iso*-$PGF_{2\alpha}$ and 11-dehydro-TXB_2, and by the downregulation of these metabolites following weight loss in obesity. These abnormalities leading to TXA_2-dependent platelet activation appeared to be driven by inflammatory triggers that were, at least in part, downregulated following a successful weight loss program. Thus, these results suggest that in abdominal obesity, low-grade inflammation may trigger thromboxane-dependent platelet activation mediated, at least in part, through enhanced lipid peroxidation [27].

Subsequent observations by our group elucidated the concept that insulin resistance *per se* is a major determinant of increased platelet activation in obesity, independently of underlying inflammation [28]. Successful weight loss or the insulin-sensitizer pioglitazone were associated with a concomitant improvement in insulin sensitivity and platelet activation. These findings are consistent with the evidence that interventions such as caloric restriction, exercise and insulin sensitizing agents may modulate most of the abnormalities predisposing to atherothrombosis in the metabolic syndrome.

2.2. Hyperglycemia and diabetes mellitus

2.2.1. Low-grade inflammation coupled with oxidative stress

The abnormal metabolic state that accompanies diabetes, including insulin resistance, hyperglycemia and excess free fatty acid release activates various adverse systems such as oxidative stress, AGE/RAGE system, endothelial dysfunction, eventually leading to inflammation, vasoconstriction and thrombosis.

In 1876 Ebstein showed that high doses of salicylates yielded lower glucose levels in diabetic patients, but the role of inflammation in the pathogenesis of diabetes mellitus was not immediately unravelled [reviewed in 8]. The expression of proinflammatory cytokines and other mediators, including adhesion molecules, suggests that inflammatory processes may contribute to vascular disease in diabetes. Plasma TNF-α concentration is related to insulin resistance, and it falls with dietary restriction and weight loss [29], whereas IL-6 and CRP are increased in type 1 and 2 diabetes [30,31]. All of them may induce a phenotypic change of endothelial cells and/or monocytes, leading to increased production of tissue factor (TF), the major procoagulant found in atherosclerotic plaques along with alterations in soluble coagulation and fibrinolytic factors [32].

Although the underlying mechanisms are incompletely understood, it has been postulated that oxidative stress due to chronic hyperglycemia may play an important role in the etiology of diabetic complications [33]. Hyperglycemia may induce ROS production directly via glucose metabolism and auto-oxidation and indirectly through the formation of AGE and their receptor binding. ROS may, in turn, activate other signaling molecules, such as PKC and NF-κB leading to transcription of genes encoding cytokines, growth factors and endothelial cell matrix proteins [33].

In addition to increased ROS production, plasma from patients whose diabetes is poorly controlled has less antioxidant capacity and contains increased levels of lipid hydroperoxides, and F_2-isoprostanes, only partially reversible in association with improved glycemic control [34]. We have suggested that enhanced peroxidation of arachidonic acid to form biologically active isoprostanes may represent an important biochemical link between impaired glycemic control and persistent platelet activation [34]. Moreover, biochemical signals of enhanced lipid peroxidation and platelet activation can be appreciated early at the onset of diabetes mellitus and that their variable intensity is driven, at least in part, by IL-6 production and disease duration [31].

Once established, oxidative stress may sustain a vicious circle, because it has been shown that hydrogen peroxide induces the IL-6 promoter by activating NF-κB. IL-6, in turn, could induce a prothrombotic state by enhancing thrombin-induced platelet activation [33]. Other inflammatory mediators or the immune reaction per se may represent the main triggers of enhanced lipid peroxidation and platelet activation. Indeed, ROS can promote a proinflammatory/prothrombogenic phenotype within the microvasculature by a variety of mechanisms, including the inactivation of NO, the activation of redox-sensitive transcription factors (e.g., NF-κB) that govern the expression of endothelial cell adhesion molecules (e.g., P-selectin), and the activation of enzymes (e.g., phospholipase A_2) that produce leukocyte-stimulating inflammatory mediators (e.g., platelet-activating factor). The adhesion of circulating blood cells (leukocytes, platelets) to vascular endothelium is a key element of the proinflammatory and prothrombogenic phenotype assumed by the vasculature in diabetes mellitus and other disease states that are associated with an oxidative stress.

2.2.2. *Functional read-outs of enhanced inflammation and oxidative stress: coagulative and platelet activation*

The hypothesis that alterations in platelets and endothelial damage may occur early in the diabetic state has been suggested since the early eighties with the demonstration that diabetic animals show enhanced platelet aggregation in response to several agonists, and that these alterations occur before vessel wall changes develop [35,36].

Increased platelet aggregation in diabetes mellitus was recognized already in 1965 [37]; since then many studies have demonstrated that platelet degranulation and synthesis of TXA_2 derivatives mediating further platelet activation are increased in DM [33,38].

Daví et al. had previously demonstrated enhanced thromboxane biosynthesis in type 2 diabetes and provided evidence for its platelet origin and its reduction in response to tight metabolic control [39]. Moreover, they provided evidence that the metabolic disorder rather than the attendant vascular disease is responsible for persistent platelet activation in this setting [40]. Furthermore, it was found that urinary excretion of 8-*iso*-$PGF_{2\alpha}$ was abnormally elevated in the vast majority of patients with type 2 diabetes carefully characterized for other variables potentially influencing lipid peroxidation [34]. A highly significant correlation between blood glucose and urinary 8-*iso*-$PGF_{2\alpha}$ suggested that lipid peroxidation may be, at least in part, related to the determinants of glycemic control [34]. Intensive antidiabetic treatment reduced both blood glucose levels and urinary 8-*iso*-$PGF_{2\alpha}$ excretion rates, and the average extent of this inhibition showed a remarkable good fitting with the linear relation between blood glucose and urinary 8-*iso*-$PGF_{2\alpha}$ established at baseline in type 2 diabetes patients [34]. This evidence, coupled with the observation of similar findings in type 1 diabetes, supports the hypothesis that impaired glycemic control rather the attendant macrovascular complications is responsible for enhanced formation of F_2-isoprostanes in type 2 diabetes.

Improvement of metabolic control in these patients was also accompanied by a significant reduction in 11-dehydro-TXB_2 excretion. On the basis of these findings, it was suggested that changes in the rate of arachidonate peroxidation to form biologically active *iso*-eicosanoids, such as 8-*iso*-$PGF_{2\alpha}$, may represent an important biochemical link between altered glycemic control, oxidant stress and platelet activation in type 2 diabetes [34].

We have also demonstrated that both lipid and protein oxidation are significantly elevated in patients with T2DM [40]. The strong association of F2-isoprostane formation with both urinary 11-dehydro-TXB_2 excretion rate and plasma F1+2 levels suggested that lipid peroxidation can affect platelet as well as coagulative activation, thus contributing to a pro thrombotic state in T2DM [41].

Subsequent observations by our group demonstrated thromboxane-dependent CD40L release in type 2 diabetes, by showing higher sCD40L levels in association with increased 8-*iso*-$PGF_{2\alpha}$ and 11-dehydro-TXB_2 excretion, reversible with improving metabolic control or low-dose aspirin [42]. Our findings suggest a possible vicious cycle in which inflammatory stimuli induce increased lipid peroxidation with consequent platelet activation resulting in further oxidant stress.

3. Conclusions

In conclusion, low-grade inflammation, oxidative stress, and platelet/coagulative activation appear as the mechanisms underlying the features of metabolic syndrome (Fig. 1).

A large body of clinical and experimental evidence supports the hypothesis that bioactive products of lipid peroxidation, including F_2 isoprostanes, are important transducers of the effects of metabolic and hemodynamic abnormalities associated with components

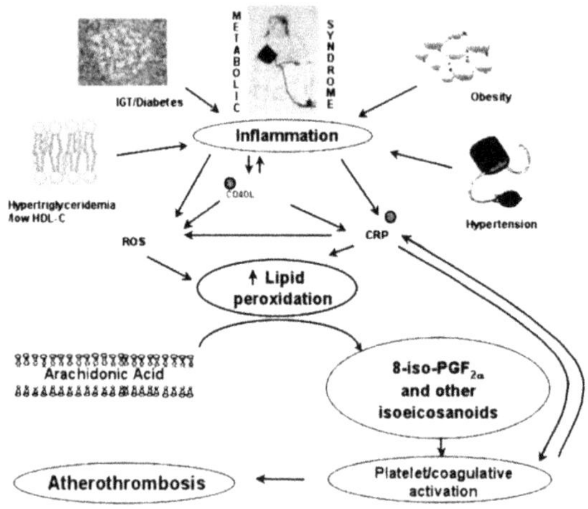

Fig. 1. Inflammation, lipid peroxidation and platelet activation are important transducers of the effects of metabolic and hemodynamic abnormalities associated with components of the metabolic syndrome into an increased risk of atherothrombosis.

of the metabolic syndrome into an increased risk of atherothrombosis. Possible vicious cycles amplify this putative cascade sustaining the susceptibility to develop accelerated atherosclerosis and atherothrombosis. The inflammatory response in each of these conditions is the link that, through ROS formation and consequent lipid peroxidation and platelet activation, brings to atherosclerosis.

Interventions addressed to interrupt this deleterious cascade are likely to provide clinical benefits in terms of modulation of adverse outcomes in patients with metabolic syndrome.

Acknowledgments

This research was supported by EC FP6 funding (LSHM-CT-2004-0050333). This publication reflects only the author's views. The Commission is not liable for any use that may be made of information herein.

References

[1] H.M. Lakka, et al., The metabolic syndrome and total and cardiovascular disease mortality in middle-aged men, JAMA 288 (2002) 2709–2716.
[2] E.S. Ford, W.H. Giles, W.H. Dietz, Prevalence of the metabolic syndrome among US adults: findings from the third National Health and Nutrition Examination Survey, JAMA 287 (2002) 356–359.
[3] B.E. Klein, R. Klein, K.E. Lee, Components of the metabolic syndrome and risk of cardiovascular disease and diabetes in beaver dam, Diabetes Care 25 (2002) 1790–1794.
[4] P. Dandona, et al., Metabolic syndrome: a comprehensive perspective based on interactions between obesity, diabetes, and inflammation, Circulation 111 (2005) 1448–1454.
[5] K.E. Wellen, G.S. Hotamisligil, Obesity-induced inflammatory changes in adipose tissue, J. Clin. Invest. 112 (2003) 1785–1788.
[6] P.M. Ridker, et al., C-reactive protein, the metabolic syndrome, and risk of incident cardiovascular events: an 8-year follow-up of 14719 initially healthy American women, Circulation 107 (2003) 391–397.

[7] S. Devaraj, D.Y. Xu, I. Jialal, C-reactive protein increases plasminogen activator inhibitor-1 expression and activity in human aortic endothelial cells: implications for the metabolic syndrome and atherothrombosis, Circulation 107 (2003) 398–404.

[8] S.E. Shoelson, J. Lee, A.B. Goldfine, Inflammation and insulin resistance, J. Clin. Invest. 116 (2006) 1793–1801.

[9] D.C. Lau, et al., Adipokines: molecular links between obesity and atherosclerosis, Am. J. Physiol.: Heart Circ. Physiol. 288 (2005) H2031–H2041.

[10] H. Kato, et al., Adiponectin acts as an endogenous antithrombotic factor, Arterioscler. Thromb. Vasc. Biol. 26 (2006) 224–230.

[11] M.R. Manigrasso, et al., Association between circulating adiponectin and IL-10 levels in android obesity: effects of weight loss, J. Clin. Endocrinol. Metab. 90 (2005) 5876–5879.

[12] M.T. Guagnano, et al., Leptin increase is associated with markers of the hemostatic system in obese healthy women, J. Thromb. Haemost. 1 (2003) 2330–2334.

[13] D. Cai, et al., Local and systemic insulin resistance resulting from hepatic activation of IKK-beta and NF-kappaB, Nat. Med. 11 (2005) 183–190.

[14] B. Albiger, et al., Toll-like receptor 9 acts at an early stage in host defence against pneumococcal infection, Cell Microbiol. 9 (2007) 633–644.

[15] S. Furukawa, et al., Increased oxidative stress in obesity and its impact on metabolic syndrome, J. Clin. Invest. 114 (2004) 1752–1761.

[16] C.K. Roberts, et al., Oxidative stress and dysregulation of NAD(P)H oxidase and antioxidant enzymes in diet-induced metabolic syndrome, Metabolism 55 (2006) 928–934.

[17] P. Meerarani, et al., Metabolic syndrome and diabetic atherothrombosis: implications in vascular complications, Curr. Mol. Med. 6 (2006) 501–514.

[18] P.H. Groop, C. Forsblom, M.C. Thomas, Mechanisms of disease: pathway-selective insulin resistance and microvascular complications of diabetes, Nat. Clin. Pract. Endocrinol. Metab. 1 (2005) 100–110.

[19] J.A. Kim, et al., Reciprocal relationships between insulin resistance and endothelial dysfunction: molecular and pathophysiological mechanisms, Circulation 113 (2006) 1888–1904.

[20] F. Angelico, et al., Enhanced soluble CD40L in patients with the metabolic syndrome: relationship with in vivo thrombin generation, Diabetologia 49 (2006) 1169–1174.

[21] V. Henn, et al., The inflammatory action of CD40 ligand (CD154) expressed on activated human platelets is temporally limited by coexpressed CD40, Blood 98 (2001) 1047–1054.

[22] G. Anfossi, M. Trovati, Pathophysiology of platelet resistance to anti-aggregating agents in insulin resistance and type 2 diabetes: implications for anti-aggregating therapy, Cardiovasc. Hematol. Agents Med. Chem. 4 (2006) 111–128.

[23] M. Romano, et al., Association of inflammation markers with impaired insulin sensitivity and coagulative activation in obese healthy women, J. Clin. Endocrinol. Metab. 88 (2003) 5321–5326.

[24] H.P. Kohler, P.J. Grant, Plasminogen-activator inhibitor type 1 and coronary artery disease, N. Engl. J. Med. 342 (2000) 1792–1801.

[25] P. Ferroni, et al., Increased PAI-1 levels in android obesity: correlation with oxidative stress, J. Thromb. Haemost. 3 (2005) 1086–1087.

[26] G. Daví, et al., Platelet activation in obese women: role of inflammation and oxidant stress, JAMA 288 (2002) 2008–2014.

[27] C. Patrono, A. Falco, G. Daví, Isoprostane formation and inhibition in atherothrombosis, Curr. Opin. Pharmacol. 5 (2005) 198–203.

[28] S. Basili, G. Pacini, M.T. Guagnano, et al., Insulin resistance as a determinant of platelet activation in obese women, J Am Coll Cardiol 48 (2006) 2531–2538.

[29] P. Dandona, et al., Tumor necrosis factor-alpha in sera of obese patients: fall with weight loss, J. Clin. Endocrinol. Metab. 83 (1998) 2907–2910.

[30] A.D. Pradhan, et al., C-reactive protein, interleukin 6, and risk of developing type 2 diabetes mellitus, JAMA 286 (2001) 327–334.

[31] G. Daví, Enhanced lipid peroxidation and platelet activation in the early phase of type 1 diabetes mellitus: role of IL-6 and disease duration, Circulation 107 (2003) 3199–3203.

[32] K. Kario, et al., Activation of tissue factor-induced coagulation and endothelial cell dysfunction in non-insulin-dependent diabetic patients with microalbuminuria, Arterioscler. Thromb. Vasc. Biol. 15 (1995) 1114–1120.

[33] P. Ferroni, et al., Platelet activation in type 2 diabetes mellitus, J. Thromb. Haemost. 2 (2004) 1282–1291.
[34] G. Daví, et al., In vivo formation of 8-*iso*-prostaglandin F_2alpha and platelet activation in diabetes mellitus: effects of improved metabolic control and vitamin E supplementation, Circulation 99 (1999) 224–229.
[35] G. Daví, P. Ferroni, Microparticles in type 2 diabetes mellitus, J. Thromb. Haemost. 3 (2005) 1166–1167.
[36] A. Strano, G. Daví, C. Patrono, In vivo platelet activation in diabetes mellitus, Semin. Thromb. Hemost. 17 (1991) 422–425.
[37] J.M. Bridges, et al., An effect of D-glucose on platelet stickiness, Lancet 1 (1965) 75–77.
[38] G. Daví, et al., Thromboxane B_2 formation and platelet sensitivity to prostacyclin in insulin-dependent and insulin-independent diabetics, Thromb. Res. 26 (1982) 359–370.
[39] G. Daví, et al., Thromboxane biosynthesis and platelet function in type II diabetes mellitus, N. Engl. J. Med. 322 (1990) 1769–1774.
[40] G. Daví, et al., Diabetes mellitus, hypercholesterolemia, and hypertension but not vascular disease per se are associated with persistent platelet activation in vivo. Evidence derived from the study of peripheral arterial disease, Circulation 96 (1997) 69–75.
[41] R. De Cristofaro, et al., Lipid and protein oxidation contribute to a prothrombotic state in patients with type 2 diabetes mellitus, J. Thromb. Haemost. 1 (2003) 250–256.
[42] F. Santilli, et al., Thromboxane-dependent CD40 ligand release in type 2 diabetes mellitus, J. Am. Coll. Cardiol. 47 (2006) 391–397.

Dyslipidemia in the Metabolic Syndrome: genes and environment

International Congress Series 1303 (2007) 85–94

ELSEVIER

www.ics-elsevier.com

Premature coronary artery disease and apolipoprotein B and apolipoprotein A-I

A.F. Ayyobi [a,b], A. Zambon [a,c], J.D. Brunzell [a,*]

[a] Department of Medicine, Division of Metabolism, Endocrinology, and Nutrition University of Washington, Seattle, WA, USA

[b] Department of Medicine, University of British Columbia, Vancouver, BC, Canada

[c] Department of Medical and Surgical Sciences, University of Padova, Padova, Italy

Abstract. Premature coronary artery disease classic risk factors primarily include increased low-density lipoprotein cholesterol (LDL-C) and decreased high-density lipoprotein cholesterol (HDL-C), as more recently shown elevated apolipoprotein B or reduced apolipoprotein A-I levels. Extensive characterization of familial and genetic dyslipidaemia has led to identification of specific defects in lipid metabolism associated with increased risk of premature coronary artery disease. Probands of these families with common genetic forms of dyslipidaemia were studied to determine if apoB or apoA-I defines genetic groups and if apoB or apoA-I levels relate to premature coronary artery disease risk. Elevated apoB was characteristic of familial hypercholesterolemia, familial combined hyperlipidaemia (FCHL and was seen in individuals with elevated Lp(a). Normal apoB levels were seen in familial hypertriglyceridaemia and in 'coronary artery disease with low-HDL cholesterol'. ApoA-I levels were found to be low in FCHL and were decreased in familial hypoalphalipoproteinemia (FHA). However, in familial hypertriglyceremia, even though HDL-C levels were low, normal apoA-I and apoB levels were seen in the absence of premature coronary artery disease. Therefore, in genetic dyslipidaemias elevated apoB levels and reduced apoA-I levels (or increased apoB/A-I ratio) differ and predict premature coronary artery disease suggesting a great potential for routine screening of apoB and apoA-I in determination of CAD risk and response to therapy.

Keywords: Premature coronary artery disease; apoA-I; apoB; sdLDL; Genetics; Dyslipidaemia; FCH; FH; Lp (a); FHTG; Hypoalphalipoproteinemia

* Corresponding author. University of Washington, Department of Medicine, Box 356426, Division of Metabolism, Endocrinology and Nutrition, Seattle, Washington 98195-6426. Tel.: +1 206 543 3470; fax: +1 206 685 3781.

E-mail address: brunzell@u.washington.edu (J.D. Brunzell).

doi:10.1016/j.ics.2007.03.019

1. Introduction

Dyslipidaemia is associated with increased risk of coronary artery disease (CAD). Although the basis of this association is well established with elevated cholesterol [1–4] and triglyceride (TG) levels [3,5–7], and low levels of high-density lipoprotein cholesterol (HDL-C) [3,4], contribution of the associated apolipoproteins (apo) to the CAD risk remains to be better defined. In fact, there are emerging studies delineating the association between apolipoproteins and CAD. Avogaro et al. [8,9], were one of the first to address the clinical relevance of apoA-I and apoB in a study of 218 survivors of myocardial infarction and 160 controls that showed apolipoproteins were as good as lipids in discriminating between the populations under the age of 50 years and better predictor of disease in the sixth to eighth decades. In addition, the bimodal distribution of total cholesterol (TC)/apoB and apoA-I/B obtained from controls and normolipemic survivors of myocardial infarction suggests that the protein moiety of lipoproteins is a better discriminator than lipids between atherosclerotic subjects and controls [8]. Work by Sniderman et al. has confirmed the clinical relevance of apoB as a better predictor of coronary atherosclerosis than plasma cholesterol [10]. Recent clinical trials using other CAD related end-points like coronary angiography, angina pectoris and nonfatal MI have been published and reviewed, with most pointing to the importance of apoB and apoA-I as risk indicators [11,12]. In fact, a meta analysis of 23 relevant studies by Thompson and Danesh showed moderately strong associations between baseline levels of each of apoA-I, apoB, and apoB/A-I and risk of CHD [13]. Observations from the INTERHEART [14], and AFCAPS/TexCAPS [15] studies, demonstrated that the single most powerful predictor of all of the routine risk factors for CAD, with a very good linear risk relation, is the apoB/apoA-I ratio, which takes into account all atherogenic (apoB) and nonatherogenic (apoA-I) lipoprotein species. This was best demonstrated in AFCAPS/TexCAPS [15], where the on-treatment low-density lipoprotein cholesterol (LDL-C) values at 1 year showed a 'gap' in cardiovascular disease risk between those taking a statin and those

Table 1
Preponderance of small dense LDL and elevated apo B in various dyslipidaemia

Lipid/Lipoprotein disorder	Elevated apo B	sdLDL	Reference
FCHL (types IIa, IIb and IV)[a]	Yes	Yes	[18]
Elevated Lp(a)	Yes	Yes	[34]
FH	Yes	No	[16,33]
FHTG	No[b]	Yes	[17]
HL deficiency	No	No	[55]
LPL deficiency	No	–[c]	[56]
Elevated hepatic lipase with central obesity	No	Yes	[40]
Type III dyslipidaemia	No	No	[57]

FCHL, familial combined hyperlipidaemia; FH, familial hypercholesterolaemia; FHTG, familial hypertriglyceridaemia, HL, hepatic lipase; LPL, lipoprotein lipase; LDL, low-density lipoprotein.

[a] FCHL is associated with variable lipid and lipoprotein phenotypes arbitrarily defined as types IIa, IIb and IV based on plasma total cholesterol and triglyceride levels.

[b] Apo B levels were in the normal range, although compared with controls, there was a small but significant increase.

[c] In patients with no lipoprotein lipase activity, no significant amount of LDL particles is detectable.

taking a placebo. This gap was entirely eliminated if the apoB/apoA-I ratio was substituted. Interestingly, the future risk was only determined by the apoB/apoA-I ratio and it made no difference what treatment group a patient was assigned to in AFCAPS/TexCAPS. Therefore, the apoB/apoA-I ratio is not only very predictive in epidemiological studies, but also predictive in prospective randomized trials.

2. Genetics of elevated apoB and premature CAD

Lipid abnormalities associated with dyslipidaemia and increased plasma levels of apoB predispose to premature CAD [16–20]. The lipid phenotypes characteristic of the genetic forms of dyslipidaemia that are associated with elevated apoB and increased risk of CAD, are characterized by abnormalities in lipoprotein levels and size and density. These genetic disorders include familial hypercholesterolemia (FH), familial combined hyperlipidaemia (FCHL) and patients with elevated Lp(a). Table 1 summarizes the major lipid/lipoprotein abnormalities that are associated with elevated apoB or prevalence of small dense LDL (sdLDL).

2.1. Familial hypercholesterolemia

FH is an autosomal disorder characterized by increased levels of total cholesterol and LDL-C, with usually normal apoA-I, HDL-C and TGs [16]. Henceforth, these excess LDL particles are of normal size and density with marked hypercholesterolemia. In patients with FH, the apoB/apoA-I ratio is usually higher than in healthy controls, due mainly to the increased apoB levels (Table 2). The FH clinical phenotype has been shown to be associated with increased coronary heart disease and premature death. Mutations in the low-density lipoprotein receptor gene (*LDLR*) can result in the FH phenotype, and there is evidence that receptor-negative mutations result in a more severe phenotype than do receptor-defective mutations. Mutations in the *apoB* gene can result in a phenotype that is clinically indistinguishable from FH, and mutations in this gene have also been shown to be associated with coronary heart disease. Preliminary research indicates that the FH phenotype is influenced by other genetic and environmental factors; however, it is not clear if these are synergistic interactions or simply additive effects [21].

Table 2
Apolipoprotein B and apo A-I levels and HDL lipid composition

	n	apo B	apo AI	B/AI	HDL-C	HDL TG/C	TG
Normal [17]	172	88	121	0.73	45	0.29	
Familial Hypoalphalipoproteinemia (FHA)[a]	87	103	108	0.97	31	0.45[b]	205
FCHL [17]	12	144	117	1.26	40	0.40	224
FHTG [17]	14	107	120	0.91	30	0.70	602

FCHL, familial combined hyperlipidaemia; FHTG, familial hypertriglyceridaemia; HDL-C, high-density lipoprotein cholesterol; HDL TG/C, HDL triglyceride–cholesterol ratio.

[a] Unpublished data from HATS [51].

[b] Data published by Cheung et al. [50].

2.2. Familial combined hyperlipidaemia

FCHL phenotypic presentation may be highly variable possibly influenced by environmental factors, resulting in clinical presentation as hypertriglyceridaemia, hypercholesterolemia, or an intermediate pictured with combined hypertriglyceridaemia and hypercholesterolemia [17]. However, an increase in apoB secretion and apoB plasma levels (Table 2), associated with small, dense, more atherogenic LDL particles [22–24], remain hallmark characteristics of FCHL [18,19]. The apoB/apoA-I ratio is usually higher than in healthy controls due mainly to the increased apoB levels, but also to a moderately decreased apoA-I. Familial combined hyperlipidaemia is associated with 1.7- to 10-fold increased risk of premature CAD [25,26]. Goldstein et al. [27] initially described FCHL in young myocardial infarction survivors (<60 years old) and found an 11% prevalence of FCHL. Others have confirmed a 10–14% prevalence of FCHL in individuals with premature heart disease [26,28]. Although the prevalence of FCHL was originally estimated to be 0.5–2.0% of the general population, a recent population-based study suggested a higher prevalence of 5.7% [29]. The underlying process in FCHL appears to be the over-secretion of apoB in lipoproteins. *In vivo* studies on lipoprotein kinetics demonstrate: (i) an increased hepatic secretion of apoB and VLDL in patients with prevalent hypertriglyceridaemia and (ii) increased LDL apoB turnover in patients with a lipid phenotype mainly characterized by hypercholesterolemia. Variable clinical lipid presentation of FCHL in patients has made their identification difficult, but the demonstration of elevated apoB and sdLDL particles has been shown to be a consistent feature across the variable lipid phenotypes [18,30]. Interestingly, available evidence suggests that apoB levels and sdLDL particles segregate independently in families with FCHL [31]. Purnell et al. [32] showed that subjects with FCHL had significantly higher apoB levels compared with age-, body mass index- and abdominal fat-matched controls. Subsequently, Hopkins et al. [29] found that most FCHL patients met the NCEP criteria for the metabolic syndrome, but abdominal adiposity and insulin resistance do not fully account for the elevated apoB levels in FCHL.

2.3. Patients with elevated Lp(a)

Other individuals with elevated apoB, who do not have FH or FCHL, may have high levels of the largely genetically controlled lipoprotein Lp(a), a dense LDL-like lipoprotein often associated with increased risk of coronary and carotid artery disease [20]. Similarly to individuals with FCHL, patients with elevated Lp(a) levels have predominantly small, dense, atherogenic LDL particles [33,34]. In the setting of persistently elevated Lp(a) concentration, data from analysis of the Familial Atherosclerosis Treatment Study (FATS) population, clearly indicated that significant LDL-C reduction was associated with reduced coronary stenosis progression and fewer cardiovascular events: these findings suggest that Lp(a) atherogenicity is somewhat modulated by plasma apoB and LDL-C levels [35]. With a substantial apoB and LDL-C reduction, persistent elevation of Lp(a) bears a reduced atherogenicity and may be no longer clinically threatening. Lp(a) has many properties in common with LDL particles, a well-established atherogenic factor for CAD. Thus, the composition of the lipid moiety of Lp (a), including its cholesteryl ester-rich core, is similar to that of LDL, and the density distribution of the lipid moiety of Lp(a) in a given subject closely mirrors that of LDL [36].

Furthermore, like LDL, each particle of Lp(a) has one molecule of apolipoprotein B-100 (apoB-100); both apoB and the lipid core are proatherogenic [37]. The protein moiety of Lp (a), apo(a), influences to a major extent metabolic and physicochemical properties of Lp(a) [38]. Lp(a) levels are particularly affected by apo(a) synthetic rate, which is subject to strong genetic regulation. Because of this strong genetic impact, Lp(a) plasma levels are affected only to a minor extent by age, sex and environmental factors [20].

3. Increased apoB, genetic forms of dyslipidaemia and response to lipid-lowering therapy in FATS

The prevalence of FCHL, FH and elevated Lp(a) has also been studied in men, aged ≤62 years, with coronary disease diagnosed by angiography and elevated levels of plasma apoB (apoB > 125 mg dl^{-1}), originally studied in the FATS, a secondary CAD prevention trial using an intensive lipid-lowering pharmacological approach [39]. About 54% of FATS probands, with elevated apoB from large and well-characterized families, were found to be affected by FCHL, whereas only 23% had FH, and 23% elevated levels of Lp(a) [33]. To be diagnosed as a patient with elevated Lp(a) the proband had to have elevated Lp(a) and apoB with no other forms of dyslipidaemia. Familial combined hyperlipidaemia appears to be the most common lipid disorder in men with CAD, younger than 62 years of age. Although no direct data are available, it is plausible that the prevalence of premature CAD in FCHL is similar in postmenopausal women.

Familial combined hyperlipidaemia is usually a challenging diagnosis as it requires study of the patient's family, a factor potentially limiting the usefulness of our findings for the practicing doctor. However, when a family study is not available, measurement of plasma apoB represents a critical surrogate parameter to identify patients with FCHL [40]. In fact, in our population of 51 middle-aged men with CAD, with high apoB (without liver, thyroid or kidney diseases), all those who did not have FH or elevated Lp(a) levels, had FCHL. Subjects with FCHL, regardless of their lipid phenotype, have increased apoB and sdLDL [18]. When a family history indicates premature CAD, but a family study is not possible, measurement of Lp(a) and apoB will add information towards choosing optimal therapy.

Patients with high apoB and sdLDL have a threefold increased risk of premature CAD [22,24], but are more responsive to a pharmacologically induced CAD improvement than individuals with large, buoyant LDL particles [41,42]. Changes in LDL buoyancy with intensive therapy are clinically important predictors of CAD angiographic outcome through a pathophysiological mechanism that recognizes the modulation of hepatic lipase activity as a key player to promote antiatherogenic changes in LDL and HDL size and density. This pathway is, in part, independent of changes in LDL-C and apoB levels [43]. Subjects with sdLDL at baseline, such as patients with FCHL or elevated Lp(a), seem to be particularly susceptible to pharmacologically induced CAD regression as compared to FH [33]. Angiographic improvement in FATS was observed in 80% of FCHL, 100% of patients with elevated Lp(a), and only 14% of patient with FH [33]. This is, at least partly accounted for by both quantitative lipoprotein changes (a significant reduction in LDL-C and apoB, and increased HDL-C), as well as antiatherogenic changes in LDL buoyancy seen in FCHL and in patients with elevated Lp(a) with lipid-lowering therapy. LDL buoyancy did not change in FH.

The concurrent presence of these two distinct metabolic pathways is crucial for modulating CAD improvement with lipid-lowering treatment [42,43].

4. Low apoA-I and hypetriglyceridaemia

4.1. Familial hypertriglyceridaemia

Familial hypertriglyceridaemia (FHTG) is an autosomal dominant disorder characterized by elevated TG levels in probands, one of their parents, and half of their siblings and children. The diagnosis is based on elevated TG levels with cholesterol levels that are usually in the normal range [17]. ApoB levels are usually normal as well as LDL-C but carried in smaller, denser particles (Table 1); HDL-C can be markedly reduced despite normal apoA-I. The apoB/apoA-I ratio is usually comparable with what is observed in healthy controls. This decrease in HDL-C involves all fractions of HDL and appears to be due to replacement of cholesterol for TG in HDL [17]; the number of HDL particles is unaffected. The increase in TG is due to hepatic secretion of very TG-rich VLDL particles [44,45]. ApoB secretion is normal, thus the number of VLDL particles is normal [44,45]. The TG-rich VLDL is associated with TG-rich LDL and HDL [17]. Familial hypertriglyceridaemia was found in the families of survivors of premature CAD in Seattle [27]. It followed a pattern of autosomal dominant inheritance with complete expression of the phenotype after the age of 20 years (complete penetrance). All affected relatives had elevated VLDL levels with high plasma TG. FHTG was a predictor of CAD in families in which the proband had premature CAD [27]. However, when families were studied where the proband did not have CAD [26] no excess of premature CAD was found in the FHTG families in contrast to the excess seen in the FCHL families. These families were restudied 20 years later [25]. There was an increase in CAD death in both FHTG and in FCHL probands over the 20 years. However, premature CAD death only occurred in the FCHL probands, whilst the CAD death in FHTG occurred at an older age.

4.2. Low apoA-I and HDL-C in cardiovascular disease

Apolipoprotein A has two major forms, apoA-I and apoA-II. ApoA-I is the major apolipoprotein associated with HDL-C. Levels of apoA-I are strongly correlated with those of HDL-C, and expression of apoA-I may be largely responsible for determining the plasma level of HDL [46]. ApoA-I also acts as a cofactor for lecithin cholesterol acyl-transferase (LCAT), a key enzyme in the reverse cholesterol transport pathway, and it is the ligand for the ATP-binding cassette (ABC) protein, ABCA1, and thereby is involved in the docking procedure by which excess cholesterol in peripheral cells is externalized to HDL [11,47] for further reverse cholesterol transport either directly or indirectly via LDL back to the liver. Additional cholesterol and phospholipids are transported to HDL by phospholipid transfer protein (PLTP) from TG-rich lipoproteins following LPL-mediated TG hydrolysis [48]. Deeb et al. in the same review discussed the potential circular but unidirectional HDL metabolism which may help to understand the role of apoA-I and HDL subspecies and their antiatherogenic properties [48].

A detailed analysis of HDL subclasses as well as apoA-I and A-II was carried out in patients with established CAD (by angiography) and low levels of HDL-C: the HDL-

Atherosclerosis Treatment Study (HATS) [49] enrolled 160 men ($n=139$; <63 years of age) and women ($n=21$; <70 years of age) with clinical coronary disease, and HDL-C of 35 mg dL^{-1} (0.91 mmol L^{-1}) or lower in men and 40 mg dL^{-1} (1.03 mmol L^{-1}) in women, LDL-C levels of 145 mg dL^{-1} (3.75 mmol L^{-1}) or lower, and TG levels below 400 mg dL^{-1} (4.52 mmol L^{-1}). Of these, 87 nondiabetic men were selected with apoB levels below 125 mg dL^{-1} to define a group of men with low-HDL-C and CAD without FCHL or diabetes. These men would appear to have familial hypoalphalipoproteinemia (FHA). We compared apoA-I, apoB, apoB/apoA-I ratio, HDL-C and TG of these 87 nondiabetic, HATS patients with the same parameters in subjects with FCHL, FHTG and healthy controls [17] (Table 2). Patients in HATS, with low-HDL-C, normal apoB and CAD by selection criteria, showed decreased apoA-I, with a slightly increased apoB/apoA-I ratio similar to that observed in FHTG, but remarkably lower than the apoB/apoA-I ratio of patients with FCHL. Moreover, in nondiabetic patients with CAD and low-HDL-C, HDL particles were modestly TG-enriched (similar to FCHL) when compared with HDL in healthy controls, but not nearly as TG-rich as HDL particles in FHTG (Table 2). Interestingly, when Genest et al. [28] looked at the type and prevalence of dyslipidaemia in 102 kindreds ($n=603$ subjects) in whom the proband had significant premature CAD documented by angiography, a similar lipid phenotype as in HATS was found to be the most common lipid profile: low-HDL-C associated with fairly normal apoB values, slightly decreased apoA-I, with a modestly elevated ApoB/apoA-I ratio, or FHA.

The two major apolipoproteins of HDL, apoA-I and apoA-II, may have contrasting effects on CVD. Human plasma contains two major HDL subclasses, those containing apoA-I and A-II, Lp(A-I, A-II), and those containing apoA-I but not A-II, Lp(A-I). There is evidence that these HDL subclasses differ in terms of their metabolism and CVD risk [49]. Cheung et al. [50] studied HDL subclasses and plasma apolipoproteins in the first 52 consecutive patients with documented cardiovascular disease and low-HDL levels randomized to participate in the HATS trial [51]. These patients had quite low cholesterol in the large, atheroprotective HDL particles (HDL_2: 0.10 mmol L^{-1}) when compared with the HDL_2-C of 0.46 mmol L^{-1} in healthy subjects, and only 20% of the total apoA-I was found in the Lp(AI) subclass of these patients when compared with 36% in this HDL subclass of healthy subjects. Thus, the lipoprotein phenotype of patients with established CAD and low HDL-C is characterized by HDLs that are slightly TG-enriched, with a reduced concentration of the cholesterol in their larger, more buoyant component HDL_2-Lp(AI) subclass, the particularly antiatherogenic HDL subspecies, as seen in FCHL, but not FHTG. Finally, a normal or slightly elevated apoB/apoA-I ratio was seen in these individuals.

In conclusion, the clinical relevance of apolipoproteins, and specifically of the apoB/apoA-I ratio, as predictor of CAD risk [11,14,15], is fully confirmed by the analysis of the familial forms of dyslipidaemia, FCHL, FH, elevated Lp(a) and low HDL-C with CAD, where genetic abnormalities in apoB and apoA-I metabolism play a crucial role in modulating the individual lipoprotein phenotype. In patients affected by these familial forms of dyslipidaemia, the apoB/apoA-I ratio is slightly to markedly increased. When the apoB/apoA-I ratio is not elevated, such as in FHTG, no excess CAD risk was observed. To this end, a recent review of CAD risk factors and lipid-lowering trials provides a compelling argument for a simple ApoB/A-I measurement which gives an accurate representation of atherogenic apoB containing lipoproteins and their physical attributes as well as the antiatherogenic potential present determined by apoA-I containing lipoproteins [52]. Thus, screening patients for apoA-I and B levels may significantly improve our ability to properly evaluate individual CAD risk beyond LDL-C measurement [53], and it will help to define and monitor the efficacy of specific lipid-lowering regimes for different types of genetic dyslipidaemia.

Acknowledgments

This study was supported by NIH grants HL-30086 and HL-64322. A.Z. was supported by a Paul Beeson Scholarship from American Federation for Aging Research. This review is based on an article by Zambon et al. [54].

References

[1] W.B. Kannel, et al., Serum cholesterol, lipoproteins, and risk of coronary heart disease—Framingham Study, Annals of Internal Medicine 74 (1) (1971) p. 1-&.
[2] J. Stamler, D. Wentworth, J.D. Neaton, Is relationship is between serum-cholesterol and risk of premature death from coronary heart-disease continuous and graded—findings in 356 222 primary screenees of the Multiple Risk Factor Intervention Trial (Mrfit), Jama-Journal of the American Medical Association 256 (20) (1986) 2823–2828.
[3] G. Walldius, et al., High apolipoprotein B, low apolipoprotein A-I, and improvement in the prediction of fatal myocardial infarction (AMORIS study): a prospective study, Lancet 358 (9298) (2001) 2026–2033.
[4] W.P. Castelli, et al., Incidence of coronary heart-disease and lipoprotein cholesterol levels—the Framingham-Study, Jama-Journal of the American Medical Association 256 (20) (1986) 2835–2838.
[5] L.A. Carlson, L.E. Bottiger, P.E. Ahfeldt, Risk-factors for myocardial-infarction in the Stockholm prospective-study—14-year follow-up focusing on the role of plasma triglycerides and cholesterol, Acta Medica Scandinavica 206 (5) (1979) 351–360.
[6] M.A. Austin, J.E. Hokanson, K.L. Edwards, Hypertriglyceridemia as a cardiovascular risk factor, American Journal of Cardiology 81 (4A) (1998) 7B–12B.
[7] J. Jeppesen, et al., Triglyceride concentration and ischemic heart disease—an eight-year follow-up in the Copenhagen Male Study, Circulation 97 (11) (1998) 1029–1036.
[8] P. Avogaro, et al., Are apolipoproteins better discriminators than lipids for atherosclerosis, Lancet 1 (8122) (1979) 901–903.
[9] P. Avogaro, et al., Relationship between apolipoproteins and chemical—components of lipoproteins in survivors of myocardial-infarction, Atherosclerosis 37 (1) (1980) 69–76.
[10] A. Sniderman, et al., Association of coronary atherosclerosis with hyperapobeta-lipoproteinemia increased protein but normal cholesterol levels in human-plasma low-density (beta)-lipoproteins, Proceedings of the National Academy of Sciences of the United States of America-Biological Sciences 77 (1) (1980) 604–608.
[11] G. Walldius, I. Jungner, Apolipoprotein B and apolipoprotein A-I: risk indicators of coronary heart disease and targets for lipid-modifying therapy, Journal of Internal Medicine 255 (2) (2004) 188–205.
[12] D.J. Rader, J.M. Hoeg, H.B. Brewer, Quantitation of plasma apolipoproteins in the primary and secondary prevention of coronary-artery disease, Annals of Internal Medicine 120 (12) (1994) 1012–1025.
[13] A. Thompson, J. Danesh, Associations between apolipoprotein B, apolipoprotein AI, the apolipoprotein B/AI ratio and coronary heart disease: a literature-based meta-analysis of prospective studies, Journal of Internal Medicine 259 (5) (2006) 481–492.
[14] S. Yusuf, et al., Effect of potentially modifiable risk factors associated with myocardial infarction in 52 countries (the INTERHEART study): case-control study, Lancet 364 (9438) (2004) 937–952.
[15] A.M. Gotto, et al., Relation between baseline and on-treatment lipid parameters and first acute major coronary events in the Air Force/Texas Coronary Atherosclerosis Prevention Study (AFCAPS/TexCAPS), Circulation 101 (5) (2000) 477–484.
[16] J.L. Goldstein, H.H. Hobbs, B.G. Brown, Familial hypercholesterolemia, in metabolic and molecular bases of inherited disease, in: C.S. Scriver, et al., (Eds.), McGraw-Hill, New York, 2001, pp. 2863–2913.

[17] J.D. Brunzell, et al., Plasma-lipoproteins in familial combined hyperlipidemia and monogenic familial hypertriglyceridemia, Journal of Lipid Research 24 (2) (1983) 147–155.
[18] A.F. Ayyobi, et al., Small, dense LDL and elevated apolipoprotein B are the common characteristics for the three major lipid phenotypes of familial combined hyperlipidemia, Arteriosclerosis, Thrombosis and Vascular Biology 23 (7) (2003) 1289–1294.
[19] J.E. Hokanson, et al., LDL physical and chemical—properties in familial combined hyperlipidemia, Arteriosclerosis, Thrombosis and Vascular Biology 15 (4) (1995) 452–459.
[20] G. Utermann, Lipoprotein (a), in: C.S. Scriver, et al., (Eds.), Metabolic and Molecular Bases of Inherited Disease, McGraw-Hill, New York, 2001, pp. 2753–2787.
[21] M.A. Austin, et al., Familial hypercholesterolemia and coronary heart disease: a HuGE association review, American Journal of Epidemiology 160 (5) (2004) 421–429.
[22] M.A. Austin, et al., Low-density lipoprotein subclass patterns and risk of myocardial-infarction, Jama-Journal of the American Medical Association 260 (13) (1988) 1917–1921.
[23] B. Lamarche, et al., Small, dense low-density lipoprotein particles as a predictor of the risk of ischemic heart disease in men—prospective results from the Quebec Cardiovascular Study, Circulation 95 (1) (1997) 69–75.
[24] A.C. St-Pierre, et al., Low-density lipoprotein subfractions and the long-term risk of ischemic heart disease in men—13-year follow-up data from the Quebec Cardiovascular Study, Arteriosclerosis, Thrombosis and Vascular Biology 25 (3) (2005) 553–559.
[25] M.A. Austin, et al., Cardiovascular disease mortality in familial forms of hypertriglyceridemia: a 20-year prospective study, Circulation 101 (24) (2000) 2777–2782.
[26] J.D. Brunzell, et al., Myocardial-infarction in familial forms of hypertriglyceridemia, Metabolism-Clinical and Experimental 25 (3) (1976) 313–320.
[27] J.L. Goldstein, et al., Hyperlipidemia in coronary heart-disease: II. Genetic analysis of lipid-levels in 176 families and delineation of a new inherited disorder, combined hyperlipidemia, Journal of Clinical Investigation 52 (7) (1973) 1544–1568.
[28] J.J. Genest, et al., Familial lipoprotein disorders in patients with premature coronary-artery disease, Circulation 85 (6) (1992) 2025–2033.
[29] P.N. Hopkins, et al., Coronary artery disease risk in familial combined-hyperlipidemia and familial hypertriglyceridemia—a case-control comparison from the National Heart, Lung, and Blood Institute Family Heart Study, Circulation 108 (5) (2003) 519–523.
[30] M.J. Veerkamp, et al., Diagnosis of familial combined hyperlipidemia based on lipid phenotype expression in 32 families—results of a 5-year follow-up study, Arteriosclerosis, Thrombosis and Vascular Biology 22 (2) (2002) 274–282.
[31] G.P. Jarvik, et al., Genetic predictors of fchl in 4 large pedigrees—influence of Apo-B level major locus predicted genotype and Ldl subclass phenotype, Arteriosclerosis and Thrombosis 14 (11) (1994) 1687–1694.
[32] J.Q. Purnell, et al., Relationship of insulin sensitivity and ApoB levels to intra-abdominal fat in subjects with familial combined hyperlipidemia, Arteriosclerosis, Thrombosis, and Vascular Biology 21 (4) (2001) 567–572.
[33] A. Zambon, et al., Genetically determined apo B levels and peak LDL density predict angiographic response to intensive lipid-lowering therapy, Journal of Internal Medicine 259 (4) (2006) 401–409.
[34] K. Nakajima, et al., Changes in plasma triglyceride levels shift lipoprotein(a) density in parallel with that of LDL independently of apolipoprotein(a) size, Arteriosclerosis, Thrombosis, and Vascular Biology 21 (7) (2001) 1238–1243.
[35] V.M.G. Maher, et al., Effects of lowering elevated ldl cholesterol on the cardiovascular risk of lipoprotein(a), Jama-Journal of the American Medical Association 74 (22) (1995) 1771–1774.
[36] D.L. Rainwater, et al., Lipid and lipoprotein factors associated with variation in Lp(a) density, Arteriosclerosis, Thrombosis, and Vascular Biology 15 (3) (1995) 313–319.
[37] D.J. Rader, S. Rosas, Management of selected lipid abnormalities—hypertriglyceridemia, low HDL cholesterol, lipoprotein(a), in thyroid and renal diseases, and post-transplantation, Medical Clinics of North America 84 (1) (2000) p. 43-+.
[38] H.H. Hobbs, A.L. White, Lipoprotein(a): intrigues and insights, Current Opinion in Lipidology 10 (3) (1999) 225–236.
[39] G. Brown, et al., Regression of coronary-artery disease as a result of intensive lipid-lowering therapy in men with high-levels of apolipoprotein-B, New England Journal of Medicine 323 (19) (1990) 1289–1298.

[40] M.C. Carr, J.D. Brunzell, Abdominal obesity and dyslipidemia in the metabolic syndrome: importance of type 2 diabetes and familial combined hyperlipidemia in coronary artery disease risk, Journal of Clinical Endocrinology and Metabolism 89 (6) (2004) 2601–2607.
[41] B.D. Miller, et al., Predominance of dense low-density lipoprotein particles predicts angiographic benefit of therapy in the Stanford coronary risk intervention project, Circulation 94 (9) (1996) 2146–2153.
[42] A. Zambon, et al., Common hepatic lipase gene promoter variant determines clinical response to intensive lipid-lowering treatment, Circulation 103 (6) (2001) 792–798.
[43] A. Zambon, et al., Evidence for a new pathophysiological mechanism for coronary artery disease regression—hepatic lipase-mediated changes in LDL density, Circulation 99 (15) (1999) 1959–1964.
[44] A. Chait, J.J. Albers, J.D. Brunzell, Very low-density lipoprotein overproduction in genetic forms of hypertriglyceridemia, European Journal of Clinical Investigation 10 (1) (1980) 17–22.
[45] A.H. Kissebah, S. Alfarsi, P.W. Adams, Integrated regulation of very low-density lipoprotein triglyceride and apolipoprotein-B kinetics in man—normolipemic subjects, familial hypertriglyceridemia and familial combined hyperlipidemia, Metabolism-Clinical and Experimental 30 (9) (1981) 856–868.
[46] R. Srivastava, N. Srivastava, High density lipoprotein, apolipoprotein A-I, and coronary artery disease, Molecular and Cellular Biochemistry 209 (1–2) (2000) 131–144.
[47] J.F. Oram, R.M. Lawn, ABCA1: the gatekeeper for eliminating excess tissue cholesterol, Journal of Lipid Research 42 (8) (2001) 1173–1179.
[48] S.S. Deeb, et al., Hepatic lipase and dyslipidemia: interactions among genetic variants, obesity, gender, and diet, Journal of Lipid Research 44 (7) (2003) 1279–1286.
[49] J.C. Fruchart, et al., Apolipoprotein a-I-containing particles and reverse cholesterol transport—evidence for connection between cholesterol efflux and atherosclerosis risk, Atherosclerosis 110 (1994) S35–S39.
[50] M.C. Cheung, et al., Relationship between plasma phospholipid transfer protein activity and HDL subclasses among patients with low HDL and cardiovascular disease, Atherosclerosis 142 (1) (1999) 201–205.
[51] B.G. Brown, et al., Simvastatin and niacin, antioxidant vitamins, or the combination for the prevention of coronary disease, New England Journal of Medicine 345 (22) (2001) 1583–1592.
[52] G. Walldius, I. Jungner, The apoB/apoA-I ratio: a strong, new risk factor for cardiovascular disease and a target for lipid-lowering therapy—a review of the evidence, Journal of Internal Medicine 259 (5) (2006) 493–519.
[53] L. Lind, B. Vessby, J. Sundstrom, The apolipoprotein B/AI ratio and the metabolic syndrome independently predict risk for myocardial infarction in middle-aged men, Arteriosclerosis, Thrombosis, and Vascular Biology 26 (2) (2006) 406–410.
[54] A. Zambon, et al., Genetics of apolipoprotein B and apolipoprotein AI and premature coronary artery disease, Journal of Internal Medicine 259 (5) (2006) 473–480.
[55] A. Zambon, In vivo evidence of a role for hepatic lipase in human apoB-containing lipoprotein metabolism, independent of its lipolytic activity, Journal of Lipid Research 41 (12) (2000) 2094–2099.
[56] A. Zambon, Prevention of raised low-density-lipoprotein cholesterol in a patient with familial hypercholesterolemia and lipoprotein-lipase deficiency, Lancet 341 (8853) (1993) 1119–1121.
[57] A. Chait, et al., Impaired very low-density lipoprotein and triglyceride removal in broad beta disease—comparison with endogenous hypertriglyceridemia, Metabolism-Clinical and Experimental 27 (9) (1978) 1055–1066.

International Congress Series 1303 (2007) 95 – 102

ELSEVIER

www.ics-elsevier.com

The role of genetic predisposition and biomarkers in atherosclerosis

Gerd Assmann [a,b,*], Helmut Schulte [a], Udo Seedorf [a]

[a] *Leibniz-Institute of Arteriosclerosis Research, University of Münster, Domagkstrasse 3, Münster 48149, Germany*

[b] *Institute of Clinical Chemistry and Laboratory Medicine, University of Münster, Münster, Germany*

Abstract. It may be expected that new risk factors emerging from research on biomarkers and SNPs will provide more precise and personalized approaches to prevent and treat cardiovascular disease. They will be particularly useful for a better prognosis in first-degree relatives of patients with major implications on preventive medicine. Most importantly, these new risk factors will lead to better understand why more than 60% of all MIs occur in individuals classified as being at low or intermediate risk according to the currently used risk algorithms. Finally, these fascinating developments have the promising potential to provide new insights into molecular mechanisms leading to atherosclerosis and thus may provide important contributions to the development of highly specific new drugs to treat coronary heart disease, myocardial infarction and stroke.

Keywords: Coronary heart disease; Risk; Stroke; Myocardial infarction; Epidemiology; Single nucleotide polymorphism; Genetic predisposition

---

1. Introduction

Over the past approximately 10 years, the concept of overall or "global" risk which combines information on as many independent risk factors as possible has led to significant improvements of risk assessment for cardiovascular disease (CVD). The concept has played an important role in the development of effective treatment and preventive strategies which are widely applied in current clinical practice. Further optimization is primarily aimed at more individualized risk stratification strategies which take advantage from recent progress in the

* Corresponding author. Leibniz-Institute of Arteriosclerosis Research, University of the Minister, Domagkstrasse 3, Münster 48149, Germany. Tel.: +49 251 8347222; fax: +49 251 8347225.

E-mail address: assmann@uni-muenster.de (G. Assmann).

doi:10.1016/j.ics.2007.03.001

areas of genetics, biomarkers and bioinformatics. The aim of the present review is to present some of the approaches to assess risk of myocardial infarction and stroke that have been developed in Münster as part of the Prospective Cardiovascular Münster (PROCAM) study. Another section of this review deals with the identification and prospective validation of CVD risk-related single-nucleotide polymorphisms (SNPs) on a genome-wide scale, while the final section provides an overview on progress in the rapidly developing field of CVD-related biomarkers.

2. Risk assessment of myocardial infarction in PROCAM

2.1. The PROCAM study

The objective of the PROCAM Study is to identify the common risk factors that contribute to CVD by following its development over a long period of time in individuals who have not yet developed notable symptoms of CVD or suffered a myocardial infarction or stroke. The study design has been published [1,2]. Since the beginning of the study in 1979 more than 43,000 employees of companies and government authorities in the region of Westfalia and the northern Ruhr Valley region of Germany have participated in the study. Examinations at study entry include a case history using standardized questionnaires, measurement of blood pressure and anthropometric data, a resting electrocardiogram, and collection of a blood sample after a 12-h fast for the determination of more than 20 laboratory parameters. Following the initial examination, questionnaires are sent to all participants every 2nd year and the initial examination is repeated after 6–7 years. If a participant has died or developed disease, all relevant records, including death certificates, hospital records and records from the attending physicians, are reviewed by a Critical Event Committee at regular intervals to verify the

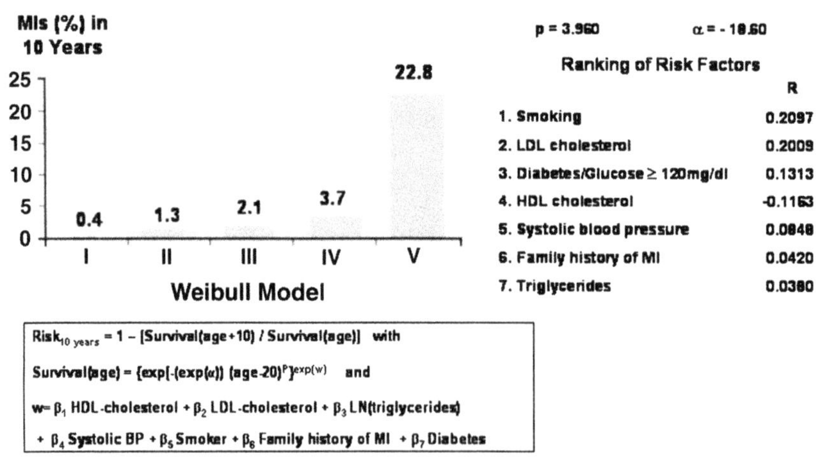

Fig. 1. The PROCAM risk algorithm for men (Weibull model). Shown are incidences of major coronary events (given in % within 10 years of follow-up) in each of the five quintiles of global risk as derived from the Weibull model for men. The evaluation is based on 462 fatal and nonfatal myocardial infarctions observed in 18,460 men aged 35–65 years and includes the independent variables age, systolic blood pressure, LDL cholesterol, HDL cholesterol, triglycerides, diabetes mellitus, smoking, and family history of CVD.

diagnoses or causes of death. Nonfatal myocardial infarction, fatal myocardial infarction, and sudden cardiac death are defined as "major coronary events" and considered endpoints. This is in contrast to other studies, notably the Framingham study, which also include softer endpoints such as new occurrence of angina pectoris. The most recent evaluation of the PROCAM study is based on 10 years follow-up of 18,460 men and 8515 women aged 35–65 years. 462 nonfatal MIs and CHD deaths occurred in men and 49 in women within the 10-year follow-up period. In addition, 83 men and 16 women suffered a cerebrovascular event while 802 men and 216 women died from other causes, mostly malignant neoplasms (men: 433, women: 123).

2.2. *Cox proportional hazards model, Weibull model, scoring schemes and neural networks*

The original PROCAM risk algorithm was constructed using the Cox proportional hazards model which has several advantages over other techniques such as logistic regression analysis: it accounts for variable duration of follow-up, censoring of subjects, proportionality of event occurrence, and time-to-event [2,3]. A pocket risk calculator basing on the PROCAM risk algorithm has been developed and widely distributed among physicians in Germany and elsewhere. Moreover, the algorithm has been implemented on websites in the Internet at www.chd-taskforce.de and www.assmann-stiftung.de. In order to further propagate its use in clinical practice, the Cox proportional hazard algorithm was also transformed into a simple scoring

Table 1
PROCAM risk score (Weibull model for men)

LDL(mg/dl)/	Cholesterol points	HDL (mg/dl)/	Cholesterol points	Syst. BP (mmHg)/	points	Smoker/	points	Family History/	points
≤ 100/	0	≤ 35/	11	<110/	0	No	0	No	0
101–105/	1	36–37/	10	100–119/	1	Yes	12	Yes	5
106–110/	2	38–39/	9	120–129/	2				
111–115/	3	40–41/	8	130–139/	3				
116–120/	4	42–43/	7	140–149/	4				
121–125/	5	44–45/	6	150–159/	5				
126–130/	6	46–47/	5	160–169/	6				
131–135/	7	48–49/	4	170–179/	7				
136–140/	8	50–51/	3	≥ 180/	8				
141–145/	9	52–53/	2						
146–150/	10	54–55/	1						
151–155/	11	>55/	0						
156–160/	12								
161–165/	13								
166–170/	14								
171–175/	15								
176–180/	16								
181–185/	17								
186–190/	18								
191–195/	19								
≥196/	20								

Triglycerides (mg/dl)/points	
<100/	0
100–149/	2
150–199/	3
≥ 200/	4

Fast. blood glucose ≥120(mg/dl) or anamnestic Diabetes/points			
Men		Women	
No/	0	No/	0
Yes/	9	Yes/	11

Age (years)	10-year risk of myocardial infarction 0–4%	5–9%	10–19%	20–29%	≥30%
25	≤71				
.					
.					
35	<66	≥ 67			
.					.
.					
65	<19	20–28	29–37	38–42	43
66	<18	19–27	28–36	37–41	42
67	<17	18–26	27–35	36–40	41
.					.
75	<10	11–19	20–27	28–33	≥ 34 Points

scheme [2]. However, since the Cox proportional hazards model depends upon the age at recruitment (20–65 years in PROCAM), the model cannot be used to accurately model the risk beyond an age of 65 years. This limitation could be overcome using a Weibull distribution including age as the time variable. The key results of the Weibull model are shown in Fig. 1 and Table 1.

A potential limitation of the Cox proportional hazards and Weibull models is their dependence on assumptions which may fail to completely reflect the complex relationships between risk factors. This obstacle could be resolved by artificial neural network analysis which proved superior to both, the Cox model and Weibull model with an area under the ROC curve of 90.2% (Fig. 2) [4].

2.3. *The PROCAM algorithm – future developments*

It is clear from the previous sections that powerful tools are now available for the objective assessment of coronary risk. These involve the assessment of global risk using risk scores or algorithms to assess the totality of a person's risk factors. Comparison of recent scores indicates that the recommendations of the ITF/IAS are most accurate at identifying high-risk individuals in European populations and therefore provide the best basis for deciding on the need for intensive therapy. These comparisons highlight the fact that even with a circumscribed geographical region such as continental Europe, significant variation of absolute risk may be seen among persons with similar risk profiles. For this reason, an algorithm derived in one population may give an incorrect estimate of absolute risk when used in another, and may require adjustment before serving as the basis for treatment decisions [5–10]. On the other hand, even the ITF/IAS guidelines have a predictive power of a positive test result (i.e., risk estimated to exceed 20% in 10 years) of not more than 32%, indicating that there is still much room for improvement of risk prediction. This conclusion is further

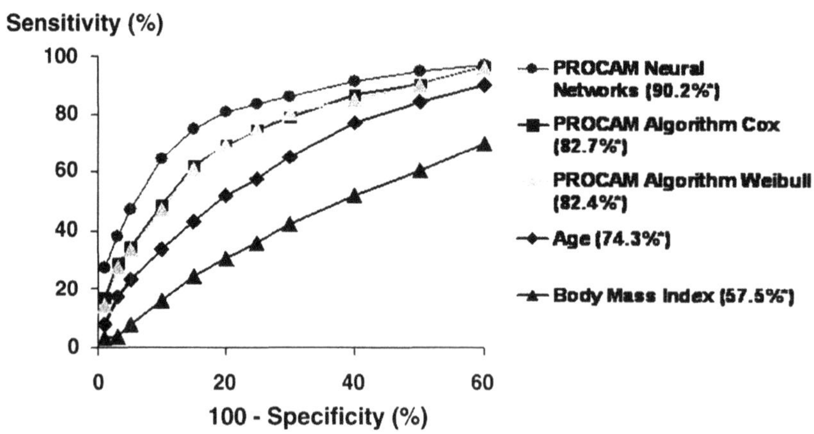

Fig. 2. Comparison of receiver operating characteristic (ROC) curves obtained for the PROCAM Cox model, the PROCAM Weibull model and neural network analysis. ROC curves obtained for age and BMI are given for comparison. Note that the area under the ROC curve is considerably larger for all three algorithms than for the individual risk factors age and BMI.

supported by the data shown in Fig. 3 which compares the prevalence of global risk figures of the PROCAM study population with the actual number of major coronary events occurring in each risk group. 36.9% of all major coronary events occur in the fraction of 7.7% of the population that is at high risk (>20% within 10 years). On the other hand almost 2/3 of all events occur in fractions of the population that are not classified as having high risk. 31.7% of all events occur in the subgroup with intermediate risk (10–20% within 10 years) and 31.4% in the low and moderate risk group (<10% within 10 years) (Fig. 3). Extrapolation of these percentage figures to the current situation in the European Union results in the enormous number of more than 900,000 fatal and about the same number of non-fatal myocardial infarctions per year that occur in patients classified as being at low to intermediate risk. Since these individuals are essentially not covered by current treatment guidelines and prevention strategies, there is an urgent need for more individualized risk stratification strategies. One particularly promising approach to reach this goal comes from current research on new genetic risk factors which will be presented in the next section.

3. The role of genetic predisposition in cardiovascular disease

3.1. Twin and linkage studies

Results obtained from twin studies support that MI and death from CHD is influenced considerably by genetic factors in men and women, particularly at younger ages [11]. With completion of the human genome sequence, it is expected that a comprehensive catalogue will soon be available of all important genetic susceptibility variants for CHD and related atherosclerotic cardiovascular disease (CVD) [12]. Although a positive family history of CHD is present in the majority of cases of premature CHD, currently, the family history of CHD has not played a central role in risk prediction and disease prevention by clinicians and public

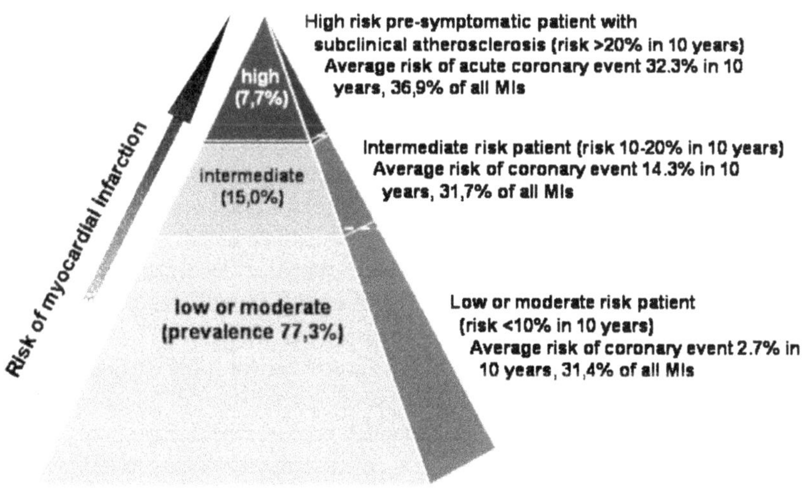

Fig. 3. Distribution of global risk categories and total number of estimated incidences of major coronary events in the population.

health professionals [13]. In cases of familial hypercholesterolemia and other rare forms of premature CVD, CHD often segregates in a Mendelian fashion. However, for most cases of premature CHD, the mode of genetic transmission in families is more complex. According to current views, both CVD and CHD are caused genetically by complex interactions among multiple genes as well as environmental and lifestyle factors which are not fully understood at present. Thus, the family history of CHD has not been incorporated along with other established risk factors such as hyperlipidemia, hypertension, and cigarette smoking in some of the widely applied multivariable risk algorithms [3], whereas the PROCAM risk algorithms does incorporate family history information [2].

Besides twin studies, considerable efforts have been taken to localise and subsequently identify genes affecting lipid levels, CVD, CHD or MI by means of genetic linkage studies and by combined linkage/association analysis. Meanwhile, genome-scans are available for diverse populations and endpoints. For example, the PROCARDIS study provided a broad linkage peak on chromosome 17 for the MI phenotype and tentative loci at chromosomes 3 and 11 with the CAD phenotype [14]. Conversely, Samani et al. observed suggestive linkage, for both CAD and MI, in a region on chromosome 2 [15]. Other genome-wide linkage scans, mainly of affected sib pairs, have mapped CHD and/or MI loci to chromosomes 1, 2, 3, 5, 12, 13, 14, and X [16–22]. However, only in a few cases has the putative underlying gene been identified [21,23]. In a recent meta-analysis, suggestive linkage was reported for HDL-C levels on 8p23.1 and 12q21.2 and for ApoAI on 1q21.3. For LDL-C and ApoB, linkage regions frequently coincided (2p24.1, 2q32.1, 19p13.2 and 19q13.31). Six of the putative QTLs replicated previous findings and fine mapping provided three maximum LOD scores mapped within 1 cM of major candidate genes, namely *APOB*, *LDLR* and *APOE*. *APOB* haplotypes explained 27% of the QTL effect observed for LDL-C on 2p24.1 [24].

3.2. Whole genome association studies

A highly promising new strategy currently taken by our group and others is to screen the entire human genome for disease-associated genetic loci by performing whole genome case–control association studies with marker sets of very high density (i.e. the 500K MendelArray marker sets developed by Affymetrix). Such studies are preferably performed with a multistage study design to reduce the amount of genotyping required without sacrificing power [25]. In the first stage, the full set of SNPs is genotyped in a fraction of samples, and a liberal *p*-value threshold is used to identify a subset of SNPs with putative associations. In the subsequent stages, the SNPs identified from the first stage are re-tested in populations that are larger. The results of the validation studies are then used to distinguish the fraction of true-positive associations identified in stage 1 from the many false-positive results that occur by chance.

Following this approach, we genotyped 213 MI cases and 213 carefully matched PROCAM controls for more than 500,000 SNPs employing the Affymetrix 500K MendelArray marker sets. More than 20,000 SNPs were significantly associated with the MI phenotype in the first stage of a three-step whole genome association study on myocardial infarction. Of the more than 20,000 significant SNPs from stage 1, a little more than 9000 were located in significant haplotypes and after further reduction of the number of SNPs by selecting appropriate haplotype tagging SNPs, 5490 SNPs were re-tested in stage 2 in a larger cohort of 600 cases and 600 controls. This stage provided 406 SNPs which were significantly associated with the occurrence of myocardial infarction in both study stages. This set of replicated SNPs marked ~140 gene loci. Some were located within previously defined linkage regions for MI and/or CHD and may therefore help to proceed with the positional cloning of the underlying genes.

4. Biomarkers

Biomarkers are proteins, peptides, hormones or low-molecular-weight compounds that differ in concentration or other properties depending on the environment of an organism. Although it seems unlikely that new biomarkers will substantially improve the current PROCAM risk algorithms, some of them may be important in individual cases at low or intermediate risk, especially in conjunction with new genetic markers. Examples for CVD-related biomarkers which are currently considered as emerging risk factors are Lp(a), C-reactive protein (CRP), asymmetric dimethylarginine (ADMA), unusual sterols, like plant and oxysterols, and lysosphingolipids, most importantly sphingosine-1-phosphate (S1P). S1P is a bioactive lipid mediator which is present in HDL in significant quantities and exerts various actions on endothelial cells and vascular smooth muscle cells. Work from our laboratory has shown that most HDL-induced signals are mediated by HDL-associated S1P via S1P receptors which belong to the Edg-receptor family (reviewed in Assmann and Nofer [26]). S1P and HDL regulate migration, apoptosis and proliferation of endothelial cells, promote vasorelaxation via eNOS-mediated NO production in the vascular wall and act anti-inflammatory via phosphoinositide 3-kinase-mediated inhibition of ROS production. Thus, HDL/S1P downstream signalling in endothelial cells might play a critical role in the development of atherosclerosis and S1P may in fact be a useful biomarker to be incorporated into CHD risk stratification.

References

[1] International Task Force for Prevention of Coronary Heart Disease, Pocket Guide to Prevention of Coronary Heart Disease (http://www.chd-taskforce.de/guide.htm).
[2] G. Assmann, P. Cullen, H. Schulte, Simple scoring scheme for calculating the risk of acute coronary events based on the 10-year follow-up of the prospective cardiovascular Munster (PROCAM) study, Circulation 105 (2002) 310–315.
[3] P.W. Wilson, et al., Prediction of coronary heart disease using risk factor categories, Circulation 97 (1998) 1837–1847.
[4] R. Voss, et al., Prediction of risk of coronary events in middle-aged men in the PROCAM study using neural networks, Int. J. Epidemiol. 31 (2002) 1253–1262.
[5] H.W. Hense, et al., Framingham risk function overestimates risk of coronary heart disease in men and women from Germany – results from the MONICA Augsburg and the PROCAM cohorts, Eur. Heart J. 24 (2003) 937–945.
[6] J.P. Empana, et al., Are the Framingham and PROCAM coronary heart disease risk functions applicable to different European populations? The PRIME Study, Eur. Heart J. 24 (2003) 1903–1911.
[7] J. Marrugat, et al., An adaptation of the Framingham coronary heart disease risk function to European Mediterranean areas, J. Epidemiol. Community Health 57 (2003) 634–638.
[8] A. Menotti, P.E. Puddu, M. Lanti, Comparison of the Framingham risk function-based coronary chart with risk function from an Italian population study, Eur. Heart J. 21 (2000) 365–370.
[9] I.U. Haq, et al., Is the Framingham risk function valid for northern European populations? A comparison of methods for estimating absolute coronary risk in high risk men, Heart 81 (1999) 40–46.
[10] A.F. Jones, et al., Comparative accuracy of cardiovascular risk prediction methods in primary care patients, Heart 85 (2001) 37–43.

[11] M.E. Marenberg, et al., Genetic susceptibility to death from coronary heart disease in a study of twins, N. Engl. J. Med. 330 (1994) 1041–1046.
[12] E. Guttmacher, F.S. Collins, Welcome to the genomic era, N. Engl. J. Med. 349 (2003) 996–998.
[13] R.R. Williams, et al., Usefulness of cardiovascular family history data for population-based preventive medicine and medical research (the Health Family Tree Study and the NHLBI Family Heart Study), Am. J. Cardiol. 87 (2001) 129–135.
[14] M. Farrall, et al., Genome-wide mapping of susceptibility to coronary artery disease identifies a novel replicated locus on chromosome 17, PLoS Genet. 2 (2006) e72.
[15] N.J. Samani, et al., BHF Family Heart Study Research Group, A genomewide linkage study of 1,933 families affected by premature coronary artery disease: The British Heart Foundation (BHF) Family Heart Study, Am. J. Hum. Genet. 77 (2005) 1011–1020.
[16] P. Pajukanta, et al., Two loci on chromosomes 2 and X for premature coronary heart disease identified in early- and late-settlement populations of Finland, Am. J. Hum. Genet. 67 (2000) 1481–1493.
[17] S. Francke, et al., A genome-wide scan for coronary heart disease suggests in Indo-Mauritians a susceptibility locus on chromosome 16p13 and replicates linkage with the metabolic syndrome on 3q27, Hum. Mol. Genet. 10 (2001) 2751–2765.
[18] U. Broeckel, et al., A comprehensive linkage analysis for myocardial infarction and its related risk factors, Nat. Genet. 30 (2002) 210–214.
[19] S.B. Harrap, et al., Genome-wide linkage analysis of the acute coronary syndrome suggests a locus on chromosome 2, Arterioscler. Thromb. Vasc. Biol. 22 (2002) 874–878.
[20] E.R. Hauser, et al., A genomewide scan for early-onset coronary artery disease in 438 families: the GENECARD Study, Am. J. Hum. Genet. 75 (2004) 436–447.
[21] A. Helgadottir, et al., The gene encoding 5-lipoxygenase activating protein confers risk of myocardial infarction and stroke, Nat. Genet. 36 (2004) 233–239.
[22] L. Wang, et al., Mutation of MEF2A in an inherited disorder with features of coronary artery disease, Science 302 (2003) 1578–1581.
[23] A. Helgadottir, et al., A variant of the gene encoding leukotriene A4 hydrolase confers ethnicity-specific risk of myocardial infarction, Nat. Genet. 38 (2006) 68–74.
[24] B.T. Heijmans, et al., Meta-analysis of four new genome scans for lipid parameters and analysis of positional candidates in positive linkage regions, Eur. J. Hum. Genet. 13 (2005) 1143–1153.
[25] J.N. Hirschhorn, M.J. Daly, Genome-wide association studies for common diseases and complex traits, Nat. Rev., Genet. 6 (2005) 95–108.
[26] G. Assmann, J.R. Nofer, Atheroprotective effects of high-density lipoproteins, Annu. Rev. Med. 54 (2003) 321–341.

International Congress Series 1303 (2007) 103–110
www.ics-elsevier.com

The anti-atherogenic properties of HDL particles

G. Zuliani *, G.B. Vigna, R. Fellin

Department of Clinical and Experimental Medicine, Section of Internal Medicine, Gerontology and Geriatrics, University of Ferrara, Italy

Abstract. High density lipoproteins (HDLs) are a class of lipoproteins characterized by small diameter and high density. Epidemiological studies have demonstrated that HDL cholesterol levels are inversely and independently related to the incidence of coronary heart disease. The mechanisms involved in HDL protection against atherosclerosis are uncertain, but the beneficial effect of HDLs might be the consequence of its properties. The best known of them is related to the "reverse cholesterol transport", i.e. the transfer of cholesterol from non-hepatic cells to the liver. Second, HDLs exert anti-inflammatory activity by inhibiting the expression of adhesion molecules by endothelial cells and the subsequent transmigration of monocytes. Third, HDLs have antioxidant activity through the anti-oxidative properties of apoprotein A-I, and the presence of enzymes such as paraoxonase, glutathione-peroxidase, and PAF acetylhydrolase. Fourth, HDLs display an anti-thrombotic effect by inhibiting platelets aggregation, reducing von Willebrand factor levels, and enhancing the activity of activated protein C and S. Fifth, HDLs have a beneficial effect on endothelial function by activating endothelial NO synthase and enhancing NO release. Finally, high HDL-C has been associated with "longevity syndrome" while low HDL-C has been related to the "frailty syndrome", suggesting a possible role of HDL in the phenomenon of successful aging.

Keywords: HDL; Cholesterol; Atherosclerosis; Endothelium; Inflammation

1. Introduction

High-density lipoprotein (HDL) encopasses a class of heterogeneous lipoproteins which have in common high density (> 1.063 g/mL), small size (diameter between 5 and 17 nm),

* Corresponding author. Tel.: +39 0532 247409; fax: +39 +0532 210884.
E-mail address: gzuliani@hotmail.com (G. Zuliani).

0531-5131/
doi:10.1016/j.ics.2007.04.003

and absence of apoprotein B. On average, lipids constitute about 50% of the total mass of HDL (30% phospholipids, 10–20% cholesterol, and 5% triglycerides). HDL particles also contain a large amount of apolipoproteins (principally apo A-I and apo A-II), and some enzymes which are probably relevant to metabolic pathways and anti-atherogenic properties of these particles.

A large number of epidemiological studies have demonstrated that HDL cholesterol (HDL-C) levels are inversely correlated with coronary heart disease (CHD). In particular, both the Framingham study and the PROCAM study show that low HDL plasma levels are strongly associated with higher incidence of CHD, independently of low-density lipoprotein cholesterol (LDL-C) levels [1,2]. Moreover, it has been reported that low HDL-C might be the most prevalent lipid abnormality (about 36%) in men affected by CHD [3].

Nevertheless, contrary to LDL-C, a cause–effect relationship between low HDL-C values and CHD incidence has not been demonstrated for certain. As a matter of fact, the U-shaped association between HDL-C and CHD, and the strong the association of low HDL-C with both metabolic syndrome and systemic inflammation do not support a causal association [4].

Despite these uncertainty, the inverse relationship between HDL-C and cardiovascular risk is supported by several anti-atherogenic properties of these particles (Table 1) including: (1) the reverse cholesterol transport; (2) the anti-inflammatory and anti-oxidant activity; (3) the anti-thrombotic activity and the endothelial protection exerted by HDL particles. Moreover, the association between HDL-C levels and longevity and/or good functional status suggests the hypothesis of a role of this lipoprotein in the phenomenon of successful aging (i.e. aging without chronic diseases and functional impairment).

Table 1
The principal anti-atherosclerotic properties of HDL particles

Reverse cholesterol transport
• Transport cholesterol from peripheral tissues and macrophages to the liver for disposal into the bile
• Exchange apoproteins with other lipoproteins
Anti-inflammatory
• Inhibit the expression of adhesion molecules (e.g. VCAM, ICAM, E selectin)
• Inhibit the expression of MCP-1 in response to oxidized LDLs
• Inhibit the production and enhance the degradation of PAF
Antioxidant
• Remove hydroperoxides from LDLs by apo A-I
• Destroy lipid hydroperoxides of LDLs by paraoxonase and GPX
• Remove oxidized phospholipids from LDLs by PAF acyhydrolase
Endothelial protection
• Activate eNOS thus inducing NO production
• Enhance NO-dependent peripheral vasodilation
• Increase PGI_2 release by endothelial cells
• Inhibit in vitro the secretion of endothelin 1
Antithrombotic
• Increase the production of NO and PGI_2
• Inhibit PAF production
• Inverse correlation with vW factor plasma concentration
• Enhance the activity of protein C and S

2. The reverse cholesterol transport

The "reverse cholesterol transport" describes a specific process in which cholesterol is transferred from non-hepatic cells to the liver (see Fig. 1), being the only organ capable of removing cholesterol from the body through its secretion into the bile [4].

Briefly, lipid free apo A-I or nascent HDLs, produced by the liver or intestine or shed during lipolysis of triglycerides (TG) rich lipoproteins, initiate the efflux of cholesterol from cell membranes. The "gatekeeper" of this pathway is an ATP-binding cassette (ABC) transporter called ABCA1. ABC transporters are a superfamily of proteins that use ATP as a source of energy on order to transport substrates between different cellular compartments and from the cell. ABCA1 transports cellular cholesterol and phospholipids (mostly phosphatidylcholine) to cell surface-bound apolipoproteins. This protein therefore represents the first and rate-controlling step in the reverse cholesterol transport pathway.

Discoidal HDLs are then esterified by Lecithin-Cholesterol Acyl Tranferase (LCAT) becoming spherical as cholesteryl esters (CE) move to the core of the particles. The exchange of CE for TG mediated by Cholesteryl Ester Transfer Protein (CETP) moves CE to lipoprotein remnants which are cleared by the liver the apo B/apo E receptor. The joint action of CEPT and Hepatic Lipase [i.e. the transfer of CE to apo B containing lipoproteins and the hydrolysis of TG and phospholipids (PL)] leads to the formation of smaller HDLs that are the favorite ligand for scavenger receptor type B1 (SR-B1).

SR-B1 is a multi-ligand receptor (member of the CD36 proteins family) expressed by hepatocytes and steroid-hormone producing tissues, that interacts with both HDL and LDL

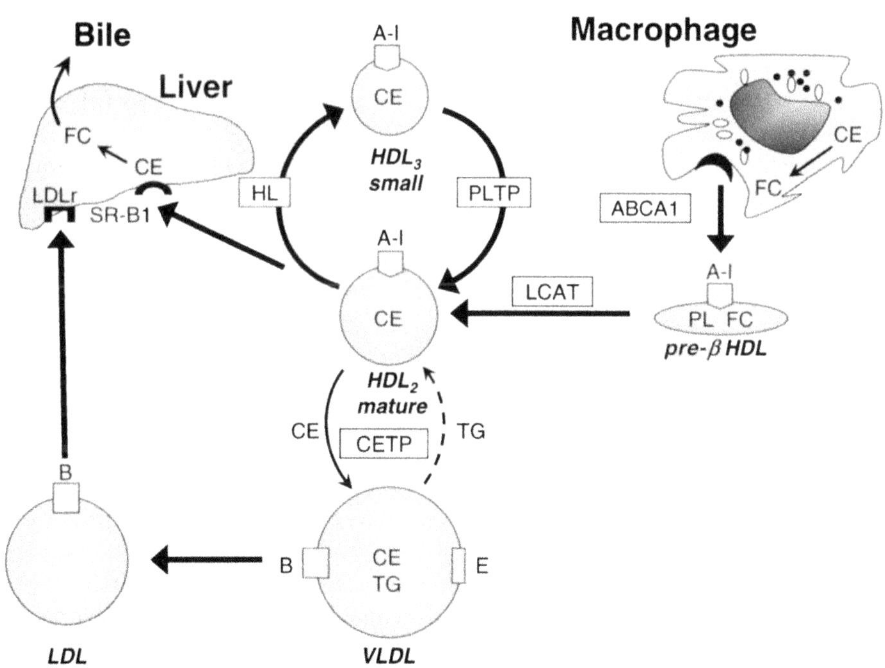

Fig. 1. The HDL mediated reverse cholesterol transport.

particles. It mediates the flux of free-cholesterol from HDLs in a bidirectional way that is depending on the cholesterol gradient; moreover, it mediates the unidirectional efflux of CE, PL and TG from HDLs, thus promoting the depletion of their lipid core. Finally, the combined action of CETP, HL, and PL transfer protein (PLTP) brings again to the formation of lipid-free apo A-I or lipid poor HDLs; of consequence, new acceptors of cellular cholesterol are perpetually regenerated.

Interestingly, it has been shown that the disruption of one or more steps in this cycle results in accelerate atherosclerosis, and this is independent from the decreasing or increasing of HDL-C plasma levels.

3. The anti-inflammatory and antioxidant actions of HDL

It has been shown that atherosclerosis (ATS) is an inflammatory disorder characterized by the progressive accumulation of macrophages and T lymphocytes in the arterial intima; this process is associated with an increase in the plasma levels of several inflammatory markers. The early step in this inflammatory disease is the adhesion of monocytes to the "dysfunctional" endothelium, mediated by adhesion molecules such as VCAM-1, ICAM-1 and E-selectin. Successively, the monocytes are recruited into the sub-endothelial space by specific chemokines such as MCP-1.

In vitro studies suggest that HDLs inhibit the expression of these adhesion molecules [5] by inhibiting endothelial sphingosine kinase; this enzyme is fundamental in the pathway by which TNF-α stimulates the nuclear translocation of NF-kb, which in turn activates the expression of adhesion molecules [5]. Furthermore, HDLs inhibit in vitro the transmigration of monocytes in response to oxidized LDLs [6], and this activity seems to be related to paraoxonase and PAF acylhydrolase transported by HDL particles [7]. HDLs also inhibit the expression of MCP-1 in response to oxidized LDLs [6], and this process has been related to paraoxonase activity.

HDLs might exert their anti-atherosclerotic activity also by reducing the phenomenon of LDL oxidation [8]. Apo A-I, the principal apoprotein of HDLs, is capable of removing lipid hydroperoxides from LDLs; successively, these products are selectively removed by liver cells. HDLs also contain enzymes such as paraoxonase 1 and 3, and GPX which are able to destroy lipid hydroperoxides that oxidize the PL of LDLs. In addition, HDLs contain other enzymes, namely PAF-acylhydrolase, that are able to remove oxidized PL.

Interestingly, during inflammation HDL-C plasma levels decrease while HDL particles change their composition by losing apo A-I, paraoxonase and PAF-acylhydrolase [7], and acquiring serum amyloid A and ceruloplasmin [7,9]. The affinity of HDLs for hepatocytes is thus reduced, while the affinity for macrophages is much increased [9]; moreover, HDLs lose the ability to protect LDLs against oxidation [7]. On the whole these changes suggest that during acute inflammation HDLs lose most of their anti-inflammatory properties while possibly becoming "pro-inflammatory".

We have recently evaluated the relationship between markers of systemic inflammation and HDL-C levels by studying a large sample of community dwelling older Italian subjects [10]. We found that increased interleukin-6 plasma levels (III vs. I tertile, OR:2.10; 1.10–3.75) are associated with low HDL-C levels, independent of a large number of confounders including the main traits of metabolic syndrome (triglycerides, fasting insulin, diabetes, hypertension, BMI, waist circumference), and life style habits (smoking, alcohol intake, physical activity). The adjusted attributable risk of low HDL-C in the "exposed group" (III tertile of IL-6) was 54%. We have thus provided the epidemiological evidence that inflammation (i.e. increased IL-6 levels) might be one of the main correlates of low HDL-C levels in the older population.

3.1. The endothelial protection and antithrombotic activity

It has been shown in the last decades that vascular endothelium is very important in the maintenance of vascular homeostasis through the production of a number of molecules that modulate hemostasis, vascular tone, and inflammatory reactions.

The injury to the endothelium, independently from the cause (e.g. hypertension, diabetes, hypercholesterolemia, smoking), produces an alteration of the endothelial physiology, the so called endothelial "dysfunction" (ED). This is considered a key early step not only in the development of the atherosclerotic lesion, but also in the progression, destabilization, and complication of the atherosclerotic plaque.

Low HDL-C is associated with the ED [11], and that elevation of HDL-C levels leads to an improvement of the ED [12].

Nitric oxide (NO) is an essential signaling molecule that induces relaxation in vascular smooth muscle cells; it is produced in the endothelial cells by a costitutive NO synthase (eNOS), and a reduction in NO bioavailability is one of the permanent features of the ED. *In vitro* HDLs, but not lipid free apo A-I, activate eNOS in cultured endothelial cell [13]; it has been proposed that the interaction of HDLs with SR-B1 modifies the membrane cholesterol distribution and morphology thus influencing eNOS activity [14]. HDLs might also serve as a carrier of bioactive lysosphingolipids that are known to fully mimic the ability of HDLs in inducing vasorelaxation. These findings are indirectly supported by *in vivo* studies that have demonstrated a positive correlation between HDL-C plasma levels and NO-dependent peripheral vasodilation in healthy individuals[14], as well as in patients with diabetes or CHD.

Prostacyclin (PGI_2) is another vasodilator produced by endothelium that acts sinergically with NO to induce vascular smooth cells relaxation. HDLs, but not dilapidated HDLs, cause a dose-dependent increase of PGI_2 release in cultured endothelial cells [15], and this is prevented by Cox inhibitors. This phenomenon might be dependent on the uptake and hydrolysis of HDL derived CE, mediated by SR-B1 [14]. HDLs also upregulate the basal and cytokine-induced expression of Cox 2 through a mechanism that is independent of NF-kb activation [16].

Interestingly, HDLs inhibit the *in vitro* the secretion of endothelin 1, a potent vasoconstrictor peptide that binds to specific receptors to reverse the response to NO, in endothelial cells [17].

Another interesting property of HDLs is their powerful antithrombotic activity. This action is mediated by the over-mentioned increase in the production of NO and PGI_2 (both inhibit platelet aggregation), but also by a reduction of PAF production by the endothelial cells [18]. Indeed, it is known that HDLs transport both PAF acylhydrolase and other enzymes, such as LCAT and paraoxonase, which could degrade PAF. Furthermore, plasma concentrations of von Willebrand factor, a protein playing an essential role in platelets adhesion and aggregation, are inversely correlated with plasma HDL-C levels.

On the whole, HDLs seem to exert a beneficial effect on endothelium function by modulating the activity and/or production of a number of molecules (NO, PGI_2, endothelin, PAF, vWF), and affecting vascular tone and thrombogenicity.

Finally, HDLs may beneficially influence the hemostatic balance; as a matter of fact, a positive correlation between HDL-C and TFPI (tissue factor pathway inhibitor) plasma levels has been reported; moreover, HDLs might also enhance the anticoagulant activity of activate protein C and S [14].

3.2. HDL, longevity, and successful aging

Since the early publications of Glueck et al. [19,20] increased levels of HDL-C (hyperalpha lipoproteinemia) and reduced levels of LDL-C (hypo-beta lipoproteinemia) had been associated with longevity in selected pedigree; these findings were justified by the anti-atherosclerotic lipid profile typical of these particular subjects and to the low incidence of myocardial infarction.

Epidemiological data from the Framingham successively showed that older individuals who subsequently become "healthy" octogenarias (i.e. without CHD and stroke) were not characterized by high HDL-C or low LDL-C levels; on the contrary they were exceedingly unlikely to have low HDL-C levels [21]. Similar data emerged also from the val Vibrata Aging Study; in this sample of Italian population, free-living healthy octo-nonagenarians (free from CHD and stroke) were characterized by a very low prevalence of low HDL-C (3.9%) in face of a high prevalence of high LDL-C (25%). Interestingly, in the same population we found that, for the same level of total cholesterol, HDL-C was significantly reduced in disabled compared to free-living older individuals [22]. The latter observation suggested the existence of an association between HDL-C and health status and/or functional impairment in the elderly. This finding was successively confirmed in a different population [23]; in the I.R.A. study we demonstrated that low HDL-C was independently associated with disability and, most important, that low HDL-C independently predicted the 2 years worsening in functional status. The strength of the association between HDL-C and health status was successively confirmed in a large population [24]. Volpato et al. found that, among community dwelling older individuals with hypocholesterolemia and normal serum albumin, HDL-C levels discriminated two groups of subjects with intermediate (29%) or low (17%) total mortality risk.

On the whole, these data suggest the existence of a strong direct relationship between HDL-C and longevity and/or successful aging, defined as aging with a good health status

Table 2
The reported associations between HDL plasma levels and longevity /successful AGING

HDL-C and longevity-successful aging
• High HDL-C is associated with longevity in selected kindreds
• Low HDL-C is rare in older healthy individuals without functional impairment
• Low HDL-C is very frequent in older individuals with disability
• HDL-C is positively associated with physical function
• Low HDL-C predicts the worsening in functional status in older individuals
• HDL-C is inversely correlated with total mortality in older individuals with low total cholesterol levels

and without disability (see Table 2); nevertheless, it has to be underlined that, at present time, a causal relationship between HDL and longevity and/or successful aging has not been demonstrated.

References

[1] T. Gordon, et al., High identity lipoprotein as a protective factor against coronary heart disease, Am. J. Med. 62 (1977) 707–714.

[2] G. Assmann, et al., High-density lipoprotein cholesterol as a predictor of coronary heart disease risk. The PROCAM experience and pathophysiological implications for reverse cholesterol transport, Atherosclerosis (1996) S11–S20 (Suppl).

[3] J. Genest Jr., et al., Lipoprotein cholesterol, apolipoprotein A-I and B and lipoprotein (a) abnormalities in men with premature coronary artery disease, J. Am. Coll. Cardiol. 19 (1992) 792–802.

[4] A. von Eckardstein, J.-R. Nofer, G. Assmann, High density lipoprotein and arteriosclerosis. Role of cholesterol efflux and reverse cholesterol transport, Arterioscler. Thromb. Vasc. Biol. 21 (2001) 12–27.

[5] P. Xia, et al., High density lipoprotein (HDL) interrupt the sphingosine kinase signaling pathway. A possible mechanism for protection against atherosclerosis by HDL, J. Biol. Chem. 274 (1999) 33143–33147.

[6] M. Navab, et al., Monocyte transmigration induced by modification of low density lipoprotein in cocultures of human aortic wall cells is due to induction of monocyte chemotactic protein 1 synthesis and is abolished by high density lipoprotein, J. Clin. Invest. 88 (1991) 2039–2046.

[7] B.J. Van Lenten, et al., Antiinflammatory HDL becomes pro-inflammatory during acute phase response. Loss of protective effect of HDL against LDL oxidation in aortic wall cell cocultures, J. Clin. Invest. 96 (1995) 2758–2767.

[8] P.J. Barter, et al., Antiinflammatory properties of HDL, Circ. Res. 95 (2004) 764–772.

[9] R. Kisilevski, L. Subrahmanyan, Serum amyloid A changes high density lipoprotein's cellular affinity, Lab. Invest. 66 (1992) 778–785.

[10] G. Zuliani, et al., High interleukin-6 plasma levels are associated with low HDL-C levels in community dwelling older adults: the InChianti study, Atherosclerosis (in press) [Jun 18, Electronic publication ahead of print]. PMID: 16787648.

[11] N.N. Chan, H.M. Colhoun, P. Vallance, Cardiovascular risk factors as determinants of endothelium-dependent and endothelium-independent vascular reactivity in the general population, J. Am. Coll. Cardiol. 38 (2001) 1814–1820.

[12] J.T. Kuvin, et al., A novel mechanism for the beneficial vascular effects of high-density lipoprotein cholesterol: enhanced vasorelaxation and increased endothelial nitric oxide synthase expression, Am. Heart J. 144 (2002) 165–172.

[13] I.S. Yuhanna, et al., High-density lipoprotein binding to scavenger receptor-BI activates endothelial nitric oxide synthase, Nat. Med. 7 (Jul 2001) 853–857.

[14] L. Calabresi, M. Gomaraschi, G. Franceschini, Endothelial protection by high-density lipoproteins. From bench to bedside, Arterioscler. Thromb. Vasc. Biol. 23 (2003) 1724–1731.

[15] L.N. Fleisher, et al., Stimulation of arterial endothelial cell prostacyclin synthesis by high density lipoproteins, J. Biol. Chem. 257 (1982) 6653–6655.

[16] G.W. Cockerill, et al., High-density lipoproteins differentially modulate cytokine-induced expression of E-selectin and cyclooxygenase-2, Arterioscler. Thromb. Vasc. Biol. 19 (1999) 910–917.

[17] H. Unoki, J. Fan, T. Watanabe, Low-density lipoproteins modulate endothelial cells to secrete endothelin-1 in a polarized pattern: a study using a culture model system simulating arterial intima, Cell Tissue Res. 295 (1999) 89–99.

[18] J. Sugatami, et al., High-density lipoprotein inhibits the synthesis of platelet-activating factor in human vascular endothelial cells, J. Lipid Mediators Cell Signal. 13 (1996) 73–88.

[19] C.J. Glueck, et al., Longevity syndromes: familial hypobeta and familial hyperalfpha lipoproteinemia, J. Lab. Clin. Med. 88 (1976) 941–957.

[20] C.J. Glueck, et al., Hyperalpha- and hypobeta-lipoproteinemia in octogenarian kindreds, Atherosclerosis 27 (1977) 387–406.

[21] E.J. Schaefer, et al., Plasma lipoproteins in healthy octogenarians: lack of reduced high density lipoprotein cholesterol levels: results from the Framingham heart study, Metabolism 4 (1989) 293–296.
[22] G. Zuliani, et al., High-density lipoprotein cholesterol strongly discriminates between healthy free-living and disabled octo-nonagenarians. A cross sectional study, Aging Clin. Exp. Res. 9 (1997) 335–341.
[23] G. Zuliani, et al., Low levels of high-density lipoprotein cholesterol are a marker of disability in the elderly, Gerontology 45 (1999) 317–322.
[24] S. Volpato, et al., The value of serum albumin and high-density lipoprotein cholesterol in defining mortality risk in older persons with low serum cholesterol, J. Am. Geriatr. Soc. 49 (2001) 1142–1147.

The Metabolic Syndrome: the treatment of complex disease(s)

ELSEVIER

International Congress Series 1303 (2007) 113–120

www.ics-elsevier.com

Global cardiovascular risk: The benefits of a precocious, aggressive treatment strategy

Claudio Bilato, Sabino Iliceto *

Division of Cardiology, Department of Thoracic, Cardiac and Vascular Diseases, University of Padova, Via Giustiniani, 2, 35128 Padova, Italy

Abstract. Low-density lipoprotein cholesterol (LDL-C) plays a pivotal role in the pathogenesis of coronary heart disease (CHD). A considerable body of evidences supports the clinical benefit of lipid-lowering therapy in term of coronary events and cardiovascular death reduction. Based on these observations, current international guidelines indicate a LDL-C below 100–115 mg/dl as target in subjects with high cardiovascular risk. In the last years, however, new evidences have emerged, suggesting that levels of LDL-C around 50–70 mg/dl are physiologically normal and associated with a significantly lower development of atherosclerosis. For this reason, several large trials involving more than 25,000 patients with stable CHD or presenting an acute coronary syndrome have tested the hypothesis if an aggressive lipid-lowering strategy might result in better cardiovascular outcomes compared to the conventional therapy. Taken together, these studies demonstrated that, when lower levels of LDL-C is attained by high-dose lipid-lowering agents, a significant reduction of coronary events and death, and of any cardiovascular events with a favourable trend toward decreasing cardiovascular mortality can be obtained. Intensive lipid lowering strategy, therefore, provides a significant benefit over standard-dose therapy, supporting a broader use of high-dose lipid-lowering agents for patients with high global cardiovascular risk.

Keywords: Coronary heart disease; LDL-cholesterol; HMG-CoA reductase inhibitor; Lipid-lowering trial; Cardiovascular mortality

1. Introduction

Coronary heart disease (CHD) represents the most important cause of death in industrialized countries. In the last decade a substantial bodies of evidence have emerged, supporting the use of aggressive lipid modification in the prevention of CHD morbidity and

* Corresponding author. Tel.: +39 049 8211844; fax: +39 049 8761764.
E-mail address: sabino.iliceto@unipd.it (S. Iliceto).

0531-5131/
doi:10.1016/j.ics.2007.03.024

mortality. The treatment of CDH with high doses of HMG-CoA reductase inhibitors (statins) have demonstrated the benefit in reducing cardiovascular events and mortality in patients with CHD and/or with high cardiovascular risk. Despite the fact that both American and European guidelines set the target of low-density lipoprotein cholesterol (LDL-C) below 100–115 mg/dl in subjects with CHD or CHD risk equivalents (i.e. diabetes, peripheral or cerebrovascular disease, predicted 10-year CHD risk > 20%) [1,2], there is an increasing evidence suggesting that the physiological LDL-C level and the threshold for atherosclerosis development are significantly lower. Based on these observations, it has been proposed the "lower is better and physiologically normal" theory, indicating the optimal LDL-C level of 50 to 70 mg/dl [3]. Here, we briefly summarize the most compelling evidences supporting the rationale of a precocious and aggressive control of LDL-C level in reducing the cardiovascular disease burden in CHD patients or in subjects with high cardiovascular risk. In doing so, we will focus on: (1) why the current LDL-C average in industrialized countries is not optimal; (2) the relationships between LDL-C and atherosclerosis progression and (3) between LDL-C and CHD event reduction; and, finally, (4) the 'non-coronary' and unintended benefits of lowering LDL-C.

2. Current LDL-C average is not optimal

Although it is well demonstrated a linear correlation between LDL-C cholesterol and cardiovascular events and CHD mortality, a temporal trend in the incidence and prevalence of multiple cardiovascular disease risk factors has been reported among adults in the United States, with an average of total cholesterol level of 208 mg/dl (corresponding to a LDL-C of approximately 130 mg/dl), during the years 1991–1999 [4]. Among American adults, atherosclerosis is present in up to 40% to 50% of individuals by the age of 50 [5]. By contrast, subjects belonging to still hunter–gatherer populations, such as some Inuit or Pygmy tribes, showed no atherosclerosis even in individuals aged 70 and older [6]. These populations had total cholesterol level of 100 to 150 mg/dl with estimated LDL-C of about 50 to 75 mg/dl. Similarly, healthy, wild, adult primates show comparable levels of total cholesterol.

Furthermore, in spite of the demonstration of the efficacy of statin therapy in reducing CHD events and all-cause mortality among patients with baseline LDL-C ranging between 120 and 180 mg/dl and on-treatment values from 100 to 140 mg/dl [7], a considerable proportion of CHD still occur in these individuals and stronger reduction in LDL-C seems to provide a better effect in term of cardiovascular protection. In the Pravastatin or Atorvastatin Evaluation and Infection Treatment-Thrombolysis in Myocardial Infarction (PROVE IT-TIMI 22) study, for example, among patients with recent acute coronary syndrome treated with standard-dose pravastatin, the median LDL-C level achieved during treatment was 95 mg/dl, while high-dose atorvastatin group showed a median LDL-C of 62 mg/dl. After two years of follow-up, the primary end point (composite of death, myocardial infarction, unstable angina requiring hospitalization, revascularization and stroke) was significantly reduced in patients treated with atorvastatin (22.4% vs 26.3%; $p=0.005$) compared to pravastatin group, despite the fact that standard-dose therapy was able to decrease LDL-C level below the target indicated by the current guidelines [8]. Based on the evidence derived from this and other available clinical trials it has been proposed [9] that in very high risk patients, a LDL-C goal below 70 mg/dl is a therapeutic option and a reasonable clinical strategy.

3. LDL-C and atherosclerosis progression

Several statin trials have demonstrated that the level of LDL-C is directly associated with the development of the atherosclerotic disease and that the degree of reduction of LDL-C is closely related to the rate of progression/regression of the atherosclerotic plaque. Patients treated with lovastatin, for example, showed a significant reduction in term of progression of pre-existing atherosclerotic plaques and/or development of new atherosclerotic lesions as assessed by serial quantitative arteriography [10]. Likewise, in the Pravastatin Limitation of Atherosclerosis in the Coronary arteries (PLAC) I trial, pravastatin reduced the atherosclerosis progression in the coronary arteries as well as the clinical events [11]. In these studies, however, a progression of the atherosclerotic disease still occurred in the individuals treated with statins. These patients showed an on-treatment LDL-C ranging between 118 and 122 mg/dl, a level of reduction currently considered inadequate. More convincing data come from the Reversal of Atherosclerosis with Aggressive Lipid Lowering (REVERSAL) trial [12]. In this study, 654 individuals with symptomatic CHD and an angiographically-demonstrated coronary stenosis of 20% or more, were randomized to atorvastatin 80 mg daily or pravastatin 40 mg daily. During a follow-up of 18 months, the pravastatin group, with a mean LDL-C of 110 mg/dl, showed a 2.7% progression of atheroma volume, as documented by intravascular ultrasound. By contrast, patients on atorvastatin therapy experienced a more consistent decline in LDL-C reduction (−48%, corresponding to on treatment LDL-C level of 79 mg/dl) and, accordingly, a slower rate of progression (0.6%±5.1%) of atherosclerotic plaque burden. More recently, the A Study to Evaluate the Effect of Rosuvastatin on Intravascular Ultrasound-Derived Coronary Atheroma Burden (ASTEROID) has provided strong evidence on the relationship between on-treatment LDL-C level and rate of atherosclerotic progression/regression [13]. In this trial, 349 patients with angiographic evidence of CHD underwent coronary intravascular ultrasound at baseline and after 2 years of daily treatment with rosuvastatin 40 mg. Baseline mean and median LDL-C were 130.4 mg/dl and 127 mg/dl, respectively. Rosuvastatin therapy resulted in a decline of LDL-C level of more than 50%, with an on-treatment mean and median LDL-C of 60.8 mg/dl and 58 mg/dl, respectively. Coronary atherosclerosis burden was not only halted, but also virtually reduced by this very high-intensity statin treatment. The intravascular ultrasound performed after the two-year period, in fact, documented the reduction of total and percentage atheroma volume in more than 70% of the patients. From this study and other randomized placebo-controlled trials using statins for preventing atherosclerosis progression, it has been identified the threshold of LDL-C to arrest the development of atherosclerotic disease at a level of approximately 67 mg/dl [3]. Below this value, according to the data by Nissen et al. [13], it might be hypothesized a significant reduction of coronary atherosclerotic burden.

Severity of coronary artery stenosis, however, is not the major determinant of coronary event. Among patients presenting with acute myocardial infarction, for example, 68% had a coronary stenosis <50%, 18% between 50% and 70% and only 14% showed a reduction of coronary artery diameter >70% [14]. Acute coronary syndromes are the result of a multifaceted process in which inflammation and endothelial dysfunction play a pivotal role. The ability of statins to modulate atheroma composition, to correct endothelial dysfunction and to reduce the degree of inflammation are among the principal mechanisms by which these drugs exert their beneficial effects in term of reduction of coronary and cardiovascular events and mortality.

4. LDL-C and CHD event reduction

The association between LDL-C and CHD events and cardiovascular mortality is well known. Observational studies published more than twenty years ago unequivocally demonstrate that the relationships between cholesterol and risk of premature CHD death [15] and cardiovascular events [16] are positive, continuous and graded, with no definite threshold below which a lack of association between lower LDL-C and lower risk can be proven. More recently, a prospective large meta-analysis of data from 90,056 individuals in 14 randomized trials on primary and secondary cardiovascular prevention, has demonstrated that statins can safely reduce the 5-year incidence of major coronary events, coronary revascularization, and stroke, by about one fifth per mmol/L reduction in LDL-C, largely irrespective of the initial lipid profile or other presenting characteristics [7]. While it is not surprising that statins determine an overall reduction by 21% (95% CI 0.77–0.81) of any major vascular event, it is noteworthy that this beneficial effect is exerted regardless of baseline LDL-C levels. In the Heart Protection Study [17], for example, about 17% out of the 20,536 participants showed a baseline LDL-C below the 'target' value of 100 mg/dl suggested by the current guidelines. Among this subgroup of patients, a daily treatment with 40 mg of simvastatin decreased LDL-C level from 97 mg/dl to 65 mg/dl with a consequent 25% reduction in relative risk of CHD, which was similar to the benefit observed in the individuals presenting with a baseline LDL-C above 100 mg/dl.

Direct testing of the effects of a more robust lowering of LDL-C level by high-dose statins has been carried on in the last years in 4 large outcome trials involving 27,548 patients with stable CHD or presenting with an acute coronary syndrome. The already mentioned PROVE IT-TIMI 22 study [8] showed that, among patients recently hospitalized because of an acute coronary syndrome, an intensive lipid-lowering statin regimen, achieving a LDL-C substantially below current target levels, provided a better protection against death or major cardiovascular event, compared to a standard lipid lowering treatment.

The phase Z of the A to Z trial [18] enrolled 4497 patients with acute coronary syndromes who were randomized to receive 40 mg/day of simvastatin for 1 month followed by 80 mg/day thereafter (intensive strategy) or placebo for 4 months followed by 20 mg/day of simvastatin (conservative treatment). Among the patients in intensive therapy, median LDL-C level was 68 mg/dl at 1 month (while taking 40 mg/day of simvastatin) and 63 mg/day at 8 months (while taking 80 mg/day of simvastatin). The conservative strategy resulted in a median LDL-C level of 122 mg/dl during the placebo period and of 77 mg/dl at 8 months while taking 20 mg/day of simvastatin. Although the intensive strategy group experienced a significantly lower rate of cardiovascular death (4.1% vs 5.4%; hazard ratio 0.75; 95% CI 0.57–1.00; $p=0.05$), no significant differences were observed in terms of the primary end-point (composite of cardiovascular death, non fatal myocardial infarction, readmission for acute coronary syndromes and stroke) between the two groups. However, the early initiation of an aggressive simvastatin regimen resulted in a favourable trend toward reduction in major cardiovascular events (309 vs 343 patients, intensive vs conservative group, respectively). More important, when the timing of events (after the four month period) and the field of enrolment–US vs non-US countries–(considered a rough surrogate for frequency of percutaneous coronary interventions and its associated antithrombotic therapies in these patients) were considered, high doses simvastatin treatment did reduce the occurrence of the pre-specified clinical end-point [19].

The Treating New Target (TNT) trial [20] randomly assigned 10,001 patients with stable CHD and LDL-C below 130 mg/dl to 10 mg or 80 mg of atorvastatin, daily. After a median follow up of 4.9 years, the mean LDL-C levels were 77 mg/dl in 80 mg/day atorvastatin group and 101 mg/dl during treatment with 10 mg/day of atorvastatin. This difference resulted in a 22% relative reduction in risk (hazard ratio 0.78; 95% CI 0.69–0.89; $p<0.001$), defined as occurrence of death from CHD, nonfatal non-procedure-related myocardial infarction, resuscitation after cardiac arrest and fatal or nonfatal stroke. This clinical significant benefit was in part counterbalanced, however, by a greater incidence of elevated aminotransferase levels, while the overall mortality did not differ between the two groups.

The Incremental Decrease in End point through Aggressive Lipid-lowering (IDEAL) study [21] compared a treatment with high dose (80 mg/day) of atorvastatin with a conventional dose (20–40 mg/day) of simvastatin. After a follow-up period of 4.8 years, the intensive statin regimen achieved a 23-mg/dl lower LDL-C level (81 mg/dl vs 104 mg/dl) and led to an 11% trend in reduction in the primary end point (composite of CHD death, nonfatal myocardial infarction and cardiac arrest with resuscitation), which resulted not significantly different compared with conventional therapy ($p=0.07$). However, when using the primary end point of the TNT trial, which also included stroke, a significant (−13%; $p=0.02$) reduction of events was observed. Likewise, when any cardiovascular event including revascularization (primary end point of PROVE IT-TIMI 22 study) was considered, where was a significant ($p<0.001$) 16% decrease of the adverse events, which was identical to that observed in PROVE IT-TIMI 22 trial.

Taken together, these 4 large trials enrolled 27,548 patients with a baseline mean LDL-C of 130 mg/dl. The pooled analysis showed a LDL-C reduction of 22% (to a mean of 101 mg/dl) in standard-dose therapy group, whereas LDL-C declined by 42% (to a mean of 75 mg/dl) by an intensive-treatment strategy. This yielded a final difference in LDL-C of 27.5% (101 vs 75 mg/dl) between the two treatment groups, leading to a significant 16% reduction of coronary death or myocardial infarction (odds ratio 0.84; 95% CI 0.77–0.91; $p=0.00003$) as well as a significant 16% decline in coronary death or in any cardiovascular event (odds ratio 0.84; 95% CI 0.80–0.89; $p<0.0001$) [22].

During the last decade, over 100,000 patients have been randomized to statin therapy in CHD event reduction trials, both in primary and secondary prevention. When examined in aggregate, these studies show a close and direct correlation between on-treatment LDL-C and absolute risk of CHD events. Computation of the univariate regression lines correlating LDL-C with outcomes shows that the event rate is predicted to approach 0 at a LDL-C level of about 57 mg/dl in primary prevention trials and of 30 mg/dl in secondary prevention studies (Fig. 1), suggesting that, theoretically, LDL-C below these values may prevent CHD events regardless of other risk factors [3].

5. 'Non-coronary' and unintended benefits of lowering LDL-C

Considering the effects of statins on progression of atherosclerosis, is not unexpected that they can exert beneficial effects also in non-coronary districts of the vasculature. Compared to

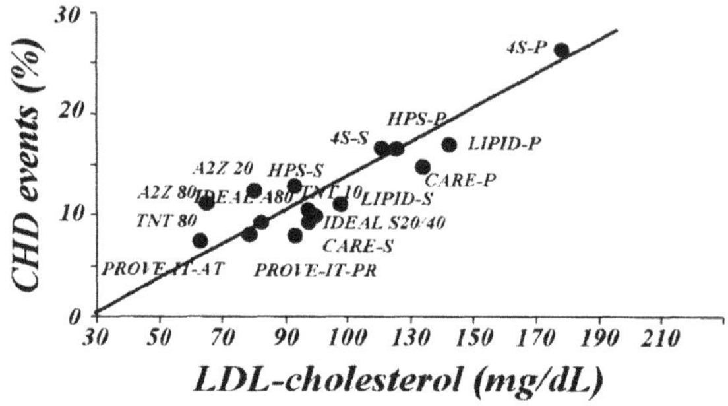

Fig. 1. Relationship between CHD events rate and LDL-C in secondary prevention trials (updated from Ref. [3]).

placebo, 5-year treatment with 40 mg/day of simvastatin determined a highly significant 25% (95% CI 15–34; $p<0.0001$) proportional reduction in the first event rate for stroke and reduced the number of transient cerebral ischemic attacks (2.0% vs 2.4%; $p=0.02$) [23]. More recently, the Stroke Prevention by Aggressive Reduction in Cholesterol Levels (SPARCL) study demonstrated that in patients with recent stroke or transient ischemic attack and without known coronary heart disease, statin was able to reduce the overall incidence of stroke and of cardiovascular events [24]. Again, the choice of an aggressive lipid-lowering treatment provides additional advantage compared to conventional therapy. The Atorvastatin vs Simvastatin on Atherosclerosis Progression (ASAP) trial [25] and the Arterial Biology for the Investigation of the Treatment effects of Reducing Cholesterol (ARBITER) study [26] demonstrated that an intensive statin therapy was able to regress carotid intima-medial thickness, whereas a moderate lipid-lowering strategy allowed for continued progression. In a sub-analysis of the TNT trial, patients treated with high-dose atorvastatin experienced a reduction in cerebrovascular events (hazard ratio 0.77; 95% CI 0.64–0.93; $p=0.007$) and stroke (hazard ratio 0.75; 95% CI 0.59–0.96; $p=0.02$), compared to subjects allocated to 10 mg/day-atorvastatin arm. This study observed that each 1-mg/dl reduction in LDL-C was associated with a 0.6% ($p=0.002$) and a 0.5% ($p=0.041$) relative risk reduction in cerebrovascular events and stroke, respectively.

Statins ameliorate, also, peripheral arterial disease-related signs and symptoms. Simvastatin prevented by 38% (95% CI 0.44–0.88; $p=0.008$) the occurrence of intermittent claudication in a sub-analysis of the Scandinavian Simvastatin Survival Study (4S) [27] and improved walking performance, ankle–brachial pressure indexes and symptoms of claudication in hypercholesterolemic patients with peripheral artery disease [28]. As for coronary and cerebrovascular events, in patients with peripheral artery disease, aggressive lipid-lowering therapy seems to produce better results in term of walking performance and ischemic-related symptoms [29].

The benefit of intensive statin therapy seems to extend also in reducing the risk of hospitalization for heart failure after an acute coronary syndrome. In a substudy of the PROVE IT-TIMI 22 [30], treatment with atorvastatin 80 mg/day resulted in a 45% (95% CI 0.35–0.85; $p=0.008$) reduction of the rate of hospitalization for heart failure independently of a recurrent myocardial infarction or prior history of heart failure, with a particular advantage among patients with elevated levels of B-type natriuretic peptide.

Finally, statin therapy has been associated with reductions in the progression of aortic stenosis [31], incidence of dementia [32], and osteoporosis-related hip and vertebral fractures [33].

6. Conclusion

According to the current available evidences, few doubts exist that aggressive lowering of LDL-C levels reduces cardiovascular events and it is expected an "official" adoption by the international guideline Committees of the new lipid targets suggested by the results of the trials mentioned above. Reducing LDL-C level below 50–70 mg/day by high-dose statin strategy seems to be practical and feasible. It must be reminded, however, that the most recently published studies did not demonstrate any difference in term of total mortality and only a trend toward decreasing cardiovascular mortality, favouring high-dose therapy. This result supports the safety of the intensive strategy (i.e, in term of potential increase in non-cardiovascular mortality). On the other hand, it suggests that, in order to achieve additional clinical benefits, not the further increase of statin dosage but the combination of statins with therapies that treat other forms of dyslipidemia (high-density lipoprotein, triglycerides, and particle size) and other mechanisms of plaque instability needs to be pursued.

References

[1] Expert panel on detection, evaluation, and treatment of high blood cholesterol in adult. Executive summary of the third report of the National Cholesterol Education Program (NCEP) expert panel on detection, evaluation, and treatment of high blood cholesterol in adult (Adult Treatment Panel III), JAMA 285 (2001) 2486–2497.

[2] S. Mayor, European society issues guidelines on cardiovascular disease, BMJ 327 (2003) 518.

[3] J.H. O'Keefe, et al., Optimal low-density lipoprotein is 50 to 70 mg/dl. Lower is better and physiologically normal, J. Am. Coll. Cardiol. 43 (2004) 2142–2146.

[4] K.J. Greenlund, et al., Trends in self-reported multiple cardiovascular disease risk factors among adults in the United States, 1991–1999, Arch. Intern. Med. 164 (2004) 181–188.

[5] F.A. Jaffer, et al., Age and sex distribution of subclinical aortic atherosclerosis: a magnetic resonance imaging examination of the Framingham Heart Study, Arterioscler. Thromb. Vasc. Biol. 22 (2002) 849–854.

[6] L. Cordain, et al., The paradoxical nature of hunter-gathered diets: meat based, yet non-atherogenic, Eur. J. Clin. Nutr. 56 (1) (2002) S42–S52.

[7] Cholesterol Treatment Trialist' (CTT) collaborators, Efficacy and safety of cholesterol-lowering treatment: prospective meta-analysis of data from 90056 participants in 14 randomised trails of statin, Lancet 366 (2005) 1267–1278.

[8] C.P. Cannon, et al., Intensive versus moderate lipid lowering with statins after acute coronary syndromes, New Engl. J. Med. 350 (2004) 1495–1504.

[9] S.M. Grundy, et al., Implication of recent clinical trials for the National Cholesterol Education Program Adult Treatment Panel III guidelines, Circulation 110 (2004) 227–239.

[10] D. Waters, et al., Effects of monotherapy with an HMG-CoA reductase inhibitor on the progression of coronary atherosclerosis as assessed by serial quantitative arteriography: the Canadian Coronary Atherosclerosis Intervention trial, Circulation 89 (1994) 959–968.

[11] B. Pitt, et al., Pravastatin limitation of atherosclerosis in the coronary arteries (PLAC I), J. Am. Coll. Cardiol. 26 (1995) 1133–1139.

[12] S. Nissen, et al., Effect of intensive compared with moderate lipid-lowering therapy on progression of coronary atherosclerosis: a randomized controlled trial, JAMA 291 (2004) 1071–1080.

[13] S.E. Nissen, et al., Effect of very high-intensity statin therapy on regression of coronary atherosclerosis: the ASTEROID trial, JAMA 295 (2006) 1556–1565.

[14] E. Falk, P.K. Shah, V. Fuster, Coronary Plaque Disruption, Circulation 92 (1995) 657–671.
[15] J. Stamler, D. Wentworth, J.D. Neaton, Is relationship between serum cholesterol and risk of premature death from coronary heart disease continuous and graded? Findings in 356,222 primary screenees of the Multiple Risk Factor Intervention Trial (MRFIT), JAMA 256 (1986) 2823–2828.
[16] W.P. Castelli, et al., Incidence of coronary heart disease and lipoprotein cholesterol levels. The Framingham Study, JAMA 256 (1986) 2835–2838.
[17] Heart Protection Study Collaborative Group, MRC/BHF Heart Protection Study of cholesterol lowering with simvastatin in 20,536 high-risk individuals: a ramdomized placebo controlled trial, Lancet 360 (2002) 7–22.
[18] J.A. de Lemos, et al., Early intensive vs a delayed conservative simvastatin strategy in patients with acute coronary syndromes. Phase Z of the A to Z trial, JAMA 292 (2004) 1307–1316.
[19] S.D. Wiviott, et al., A tale of two trials. A comparison of post-acute coronary syndrome lipid-lowering trials A to Z and PROVE IT-TIMI 22, Circulation 113 (2006) 1406–1414.
[20] J.C. LaRosa, et al., Intensive lipid lowering with atorvastatin in patients with stable coronary disease, N. Engl. J. Med. 352 (2005) 1425–1435.
[21] T.R. Pedersen, et al., High-dose atorvastatin versus usual-dose simvastatin for secondary prevention after myocardial infarction: the IDEAL study: a randomized controlled trial, JAMA 294 (2005) 2437–2445.
[22] C.P. Cannon, et al., Meta-analysis of cardiovascular outcomes trials comparing intensive versus moderate statin therapy, J. Am. Coll. Cardiol. 48 (2006) 438–445.
[23] Heart Protection Study Collaborative Group, Effects of cholesterol-lowering with simvastatin on stroke and other major vascular events in 20 536 people with cerebrovascular disease or other high-risk conditions, Lancet 363 (2004) 757–767.
[24] The Stroke Prevention by Aggressive Reduction in Cholesterol Levels Investigators, High-dose atorvastatin after stroke or transient ischemic attack, N. Engl. J. Med. 355 (2006) 549–559.
[25] T.J. Smilde, et al., Effect of aggressive versus conventional lipid-lowering on atherosclerosis progression in familial hypercholesterolemia (ASAP): a prospective, randomized, double-blind trial, Lancet 357 (2001) 577–581.
[26] A.J. Taylor, et al., ARBITER: arterial biology for the investigation of the treatment effects of reducing cholesterol: a randomized trial comparing the effects of atorvastatin and pravastatin on carotid intima medial thickness, Circulation 106 (2002) 2055–2060.
[27] T.R. Pedersen, et al., Effect of simvastatin on ischemic signs and symptoms in the Scandinavian Simvastatin Survival Study (4S), Am. J. Cardiol. 81 (1998) 333–335.
[28] S. Mondillo, et al., Effects of simvastatin on walking performance and symptoms of intermittent claudication in hypercholesterolemic patients with peripheral vascular disease, Am. J. Med. 114 (2003) 359–364.
[29] E.R. Mohler, W.R. Hiatt, M.A. Creager, Cholesterol reduction with atorvastatin improves walking distance in patients with peripheral arterial disease, Circulation 108 (2003) 1481–1486.
[30] B.M. Scirica, et al., Intensive statin therapy and the risk of hospitalization for heart failure after an acute coronary syndrome in the PROVE IT-TIMI 22 study, J. Am. Coll. Cardiol. 47 (2006) 2326–2331.
[31] M.F. Bellamy, et al., Association of cholesterol, hydroxymethylglutaryl coenzyme—A reductase inhibitor treatment, and progression of aortic stenosis in the community, J. Am. Coll. Cardiol. 4 0 (2002) 1723–1730.
[32] M. Etminan, S. Gill, A. Samii, The role of lipid-lowering drugs in cognitive function: a meta-analysis of observational studies, Pharmacotherapy 23 (2003) 726–730.
[33] B.C. Bauer, et al., Use of statins and fracture: results of four prospective studies and cumulative meta-analysis of observational studies and controlled trials, Arch. Intern. Med. 164 (2004) 146–152.

ELSEVIER

International Congress Series 1303 (2007) 121 – 128

www.ics-elsevier.com

Inhibition of synthesis and absorption of cholesterol: A new option in managing hypercholesterolemia

Liliana Grigore [b], Giuseppe Danilo Norata [a,b], Alberico L. Catapano [a,b,*]

[a] *Department of Pharmacological Sciences, University of Milan, Milan, Italy*
[b] *Center for the Study of Atherosclerosis, Bassini Hospital, Cinisello B, Italy*

Abstract. Although widely used in lipid lowering therapy, HMG CoA reductase inhibitors or statins (even when administered at high doses) are frequently insufficient to achieve guideline-recommended LDL-C goals for many patients with hypercholesterolemia in everyday clinical practice. Often over half of patients do not achieve LDL-C goal on the initial dose of statin and most of these patients do not reach goal neither after 6 months. Thus, a wide therapeutic gap exists between target LDL-C levels and those typically achieved in clinical practice. A recent and more effective therapeutic strategy, therefore, is to treat the two main sources of cholesterol simultaneously (production of cholesterol, mainly in the liver, and absorption of cholesterol in the intestine) with a complementary mechanism of action, by co-administering ezetimibe, a novel agent inhibiting cholesterol absorption, together with a statin, which inhibits cholesterol production in the liver. Ezetimibe can be effectively co-administered with any dose of any statin and, compared with single inhibition of cholesterol production, afforded by statins alone, provides consistently greater reductions in LDL-C through Dual Inhibition of both cholesterol production and absorption. Here we summarize the pivotal role of both the liver and intestine in the overall balance of cholesterol in the body and describe the clinical impact and relevance of inhibiting both sources of cholesterol either by using ezetimibe/simvastatin as a single tablet or co-administering ezetimibe together with any dose of any statin. © 2007 Published by Elsevier B.V.

Keywords: Hypercholesterolemia; Cholesterol absorption; Cholesterol biosynthesis; Ezetimibe; HMG-CoA reductase inhibitors; LDL-C

* Corresponding author. Center for the Study of Atherosclerosis, Department of Pharmacological Sciences, University of Milan, Via Balzaretti 9, 20133 Milan, Italy. Tel.: +39 02 50318302; fax: +39 20 50318386.
E-mail address: alberico.catapano@unimi.it (A.L. Catapano).

0531-5131/ © 2007 Published by Elsevier B.V.
doi:10.1016/j.ics.2007.04.004

1. Introduction

Hypercholesterolemia plays a key role in the development and progression of atherosclerosis and is a proven risk factor for coronary heart disease (CHD) [1–4]. Pharmacologic interventions to lower cholesterol levels both in primary and secondary prevention trials show a clear reduction in the incidence of CHD as well as stroke [5–11].

Although widely used in lipid lowering therapy, HMG CoA reductase inhibitors or statins (even when administered at high doses) are frequently insufficient to achieve guideline-recommended LDL-C goals for many patients with hypercholesterolemia in every day clinical practice [12]. According to a recent study, a large proportion of high-risk hyperlipidemic patients receiving statins alone were not at goal even when physicians were free to use any statin and titrate according to their professional judgment [13]. Over half (52%) of patients did not achieve LDL-C goal on the initial dose of statin, and 86% of these patients had still not reached goal after 6 months [13]. Thus, a wide therapeutic gap exists between target LDL-C levels and those typically achieved in clinical practice [14].

The therapeutic gap will undoubtedly increase in light of the recent amendments of the National Cholesterol Education Program Adult Treatment Program III (NCEP ATP III) guidelines, which recommend even more aggressive reductions in lipid levels for patients at high risk of CHD [15]. The more aggressive cholesterol treatment goals proposed by the revised guidelines call for a more advanced approach to maximize the cardiovascular benefits associated with lower LDL-C levels.

There are two main sources of cholesterol, which are similar in size: production of cholesterol, mainly in the liver, and absorption of cholesterol in the intestine [16,17]. Approximately 50% of the cholesterol pool is absorbed and recirculated through the intestine, while the remainder is excreted through the feces [16,17]. The intestinal pool is composed of both dietary, and the majority, from biliary excretion. A recent and more effective therapeutic strategy, therefore, is to treat both sources of cholesterol simultaneously with a complementary mechanism of action, by co-administering ezetimibe, a novel agent inhibiting cholesterol absorption, together with a statin, which inhibits cholesterol production in the liver [16,18,19]. This results in Dual Inhibition of both sources of cholesterol provides significantly greater LDL-C reduction and subsequent goal attainment.

Ezetimibe can be effectively co-administered with any dose of any statin and, compared with single inhibition of cholesterol production, afforded by statins alone, provides consistently greater reductions in LDL-C through Dual Inhibition of both cholesterol production and absorption [20–23]. The single product of ezetimibe/simvastatin is the first and only product to treat both sources of cholesterol through Dual Inhibition. As with ezetimibe co-administered with any dose of any statin, the single tablet of ezetimibe/simvastatin provides superior LDL-C lowering efficacy with improved LDL-C goal attainment [24–26].

Here we summarize the pivotal role of both the liver and intestine in the overall balance of cholesterol in the body and describe the clinical impact and relevance of inhibiting both sources of cholesterol either by using ezetimibe/simvastatin as a single tablet or co-administering ezetimibe together with any dose of any statin.

2. The liver and intestine: sources of cholesterol

The average adult body contains approximately 140 mg of sterol, mainly in the form of cholesterol [27]. This pool of cholesterol is derived from two major sources-synthesis of cholesterol by the liver (and extrahepatic sites) and absorption by the intestines [16,18]. Approximately 500 to 1400 mg per day of cholesterol enters the body's cholesterol pool from synthesis (500 to 1000 mg) and intestinal absorption (up to 400 mg per day) [27,28]. However, the cholesterol pool usually changes little because cholesterol input is approximately balanced by cholesterol output via excretion in bile/feces, skin excretion, steroid hormone synthesis, tissue storage, etc. [27,28].

The liver plays a central role in balancing cholesterol from all sources and also plays a pivotal role in regulating plasma LDL-C levels [29]. The hepatic pool of cholesterol is derived from local biosynthesis and from chylomicron remnants and lipoproteins. Cholesterol biosynthesis is regulated by the rate-limiting enzyme HMG CoA reductase, which catalyzes production of mevalonic acid from HMG CoA and represents the single therapeutic target for statins. Cholesterol produced by liver is either secreted in bile (principal route) or incorporated into lipoproteins (mainly LDL and VLDL) and secreted into plasma.

Intestinal cholesterol absorption represents another major route for the entry of cholesterol into the body, and, thus, this source can influence the plasma LDL-cholesterol concentration [18]. The cholesterol pool in the intestine comes from dietary cholesterol and the majority from biliary excretion. Approximately 50% of the intestinal cholesterol pool is reabsorbed by the intestines [30] and recirculated through the body (via the enterohepatic circulation), with the remainder excreted in feces.

While the precise molecular transport mechanisms of cholesterol absorption are not completely delineated, cholesterol absorption in the intestine involves a complex triphasic process (Fig. 1): intraluminal phase (digestion/hydrolysis of dietary lipids and micellar solubilization of cholesterol), membrane transport phase (cholesterol release from micelles at brush border membrane and uptake into enterocytes), and an intracellular phase (re-esterification, incorporation into nascent chylomicrons, and secretion into lymph) [30,31]. Although some cholesterol translocation across the brush border membrane occurs by passive diffusion, several sterol transporters have also been implicated in this process, including Niemann–Pick C1 like 1 protein [NPC1L1], aminopeptidase N (CD13), annexin-2/caveolin-1 (ANX2/CAV1), and ATP-binding cassette (ABC) transporters (ABCG5 and ABCG8) [31–33]. Inhibition of cholesterol absorption with novel agents such as ezetimibe has thus become an important and attractive therapeutic target, particularly since postprandial lipoproteins (cholesterol-rich chylomicron remnants) appear to be especially atherogenic, with the ability to enter the arterial wall and promote atherogenesis [34].

2.1. Treating two sources of cholesterol — cholesterol production and absorption

In the past few years, an innovative progression in cholesterol-lipid lowering therapy has occurred. We now recognize that treating both cholesterol production in the liver and absorption in the intestine, either by administering ezetimibe/simvastatin as a single tablet or co-administering ezetimibe together with any dose of statin, results in superior LDL-C-lowering efficacy and more patients achieving or getting

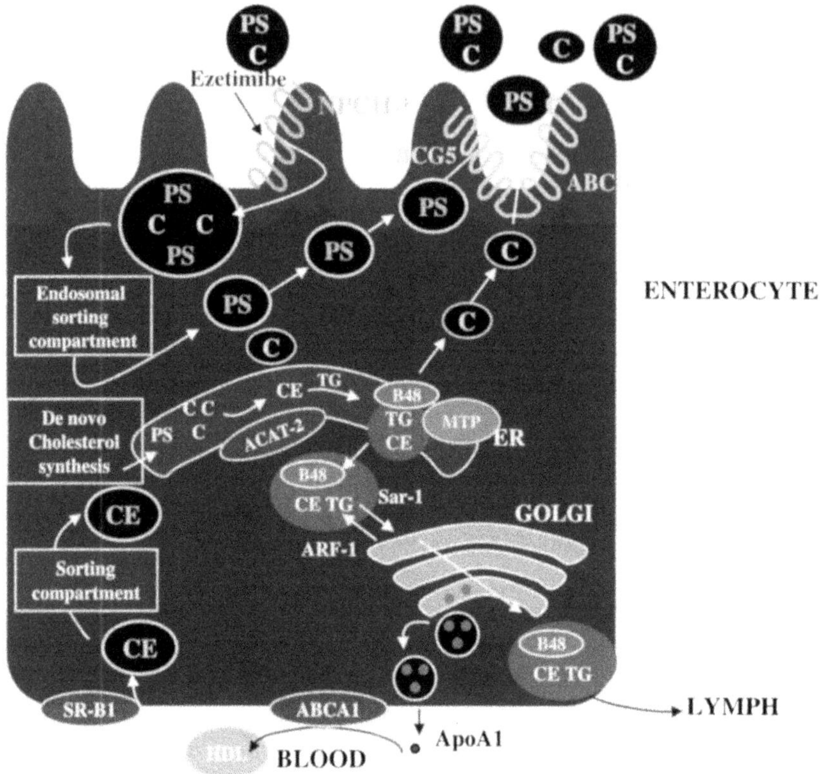

Fig. 1. Overview of the principal steps in the intestinal absorption of cholesterol (C). The intraluminal phase involves the digestion/hydrolysis of dietary lipids and micellar solubilization of cholesterol. The membrane transport phase involves cholesterol release from micelles at the brush border membrane and uptake into enterocytes via several sterol transporters, including Niemann–Pick C1 like 1 protein (NPC1L1), aminopeptidase N (CD13), and annexin-2/caveolin-1 (ANX2/CAV1). The brush border membrane also contains ATP-binding cassette (ABC) transporters (ABCG5 and ABCG8), which primarily move plant sterols and to a lesser extent cholesterol out of the enterocytes. The intracellular phase involves esterification, incorporation into nascent chylomicrons, and secretion into lymph for transport to the liver. Several enzymes and proteins within the enterocyte are involved in the intracellular phase, including acyl CoA:cholesterol acyltranserase (ACAT), which enhances intracellular cholesterol esterification, and microsomal triglyceride transfer protein (MTP), which assembles intestinal chylomicrons. Ezetimibe may inhibit cholesterol absorption by interacting with several cholesterol transport proteins present in the brush border membrane, including NPC1L1, ANX2/CAV1, and aminopeptidase N (CD13). Based on information extracted from Turley and Dietschy [18], Smart et al. [33], Kramer et al. [32], and Sudhop et al. [31].

below LDL-C treatment goals compared with inhibition of a single cholesterol source with statins alone.

Statins (e.g., fluvastatin, lovastatin, pravastatin, simvastatin, atorvastatin, and rosuvastatin) deliver only single inhibition of cholesterol production in the liver by blocking HMG-CoA reductase, the rate-limiting step in cholesterol synthesis, but do not impact intestinal cholesterol absorption [35]. As a result, hepatocytes become depleted of cholesterol and respond by increasing LDL-C clearance from the blood (via upregulation of hepatic LDL-C receptors) and decreasing entry of LDL-C into the circulation [36,37]. These actions, in turn, give rise to lower plasma LDL-C levels.

Ezetimibe is a novel, orally active, and selective inhibitor of intestinal absorption of dietary and biliary cholesterol as well as plant sterols [18,38,39]. Ezetimibe is the first in a class of lipid-lowering agents with a mechanism of action that is very different from other lipid lowering therapies, including bile acid sequestrants. By inhibiting cholesterol absorption at the level of the brush border of the intestine, ezetimibe reduces the amount of chylomicron cholesterol circulated to the liver. In response to reduced cholesterol delivery, the liver reacts by upregulating LDL-C receptors, which in turn, leads to increased clearance of cholesterol from the blood [19].

Recent studies indicate that ezetimibe may interact with the cholesterol transport protein NPC1L1 expressed in the intestine as well as in the liver and other cell types [40]. Ezetimibe may also prevent cholesterol absorption by inhibiting ANX2/CAV1, which is required for the uptake of cholesterol from micelles into enterocytes [33]. Interestingly, ezetimibe has also been shown to block the uptake of oxidized LDL by human macrophages through inhibition of both NPC1L1 and ANX2/CAV1 [41], suggesting the actions of this agent may extend beyond the intestinal epithelium. Aminopeptidase N (CD13) in the brush border membrane may represent an additional molecular target for ezetimibe. Ezetimibe has been shown to bind to aminopeptidase N thereby blocking the endocytosis of cholesterol from micelles in the intestinal lumen [32].

2.2. Impact of treating two sources of cholesterol on LDL-C-lowering efficacy and getting patients to goal

The use of two-lipid-lowering compounds (ezetimibe co-administered with a statin) with a complementary mechanism of action provides a powerful new approach to prevent and treat atherosclerosis. Treating two sources of cholesterol (rather than one source with statins alone) results in a substantially greater overall LDL-C lowering efficacy as well as in more patients attaining or getting below LDL-C goals.

2.3. Ezetimibe/simvastatin as a single tablet

Ezetimibe/simvastatin as a single tablet was superior to atorvastatin alone in reducing plasma LDL-C at every dose comparison studied, according to double-blind, randomized, forced-titration study [24]. Adult patients with hypercholesterolemia experienced significantly greater reductions in LDL-C when they received the typical starting dose of ezetimibe/simvastatin 10/20 mg (50%) compared with atorvastatin 10mg (37%) after 6 weeks of treatment ($p<0.001$). Importantly, the reduction in LDL-C levels seen with ezetimibe/simvastatin was comparable to the 50% reduction in LDL-C levels that has shown to be required for reversal of atherosclerosis, according to the Reversal of Atherosclerosis with Aggressive Lipid Lowering (REVERSAL) study [42]. In addition, ezetimibe/simvastatin resulted in significantly more patients achieving LDL-C goal (<100 mg/dl) whether compared with atorvastatin or simvastatin alone [25,26].

Further, compared with patients receiving atorvastatin alone, more patients treated with ezetimibe/simvastatin reached the more aggressive LDL-C target (<70 mg/dl), as recently recommended by the NCEP for very high-risk CHD patients [26]. Approximately 23% of patients receiving atorvastatin 40 mg alone and 36% of patients receiving atorvastatin 80 mg alone reached the optional LDL-C treatment target of < 70 mg/dl compared with 57% of patients treated with ezetimibe/simvastatin (10/40 mg) and 64% of patients receiving ezetimibe/simvastatin (10/80 mg) [45].

2.4. Co-administering ezetimibe together with a statin

In patients with hypercholesterolemia not at goal on statin therapy alone, the Ezetimibe Add-On to Statin for Effectiveness (EASE) trial [43] demonstrated that co-administering ezetimibe (10 mg) with any dose of statin reduced LDL-C levels by an additional 25% and improved LDL-C goal attainment from 20% on statin monotherapy to 71% with Dual Inhibition therapy. Similarly, co-administering ezetimibe together with ongoing statin therapy also produced a marked 25% reduction in LDL-C compared with statin alone, a reduction which resulted in significantly more patients achieving NCEP treatment goals (71.7% vs. 18.9% on statin alone, $p<0.001$) [44].

2.5. Impact of treating two sources of cholesterol on outcomes

Although treating two sources of cholesterol through Dual Inhibition provides superior LDL-C lowering efficacy with improved LDL-C goal attainment, one key clinical question remains to be addressed: Do the lower LDL-C levels achieved with Dual Inhibition of cholesterol production and absorption ultimately translate into reduced cardiovascular or renal events and a slower rate of progression of atherosclerosis? This question is currently being assessed in several major cardiovascular outcomes studies, including Ezetimibe and Simvastatin in Hypercholesterolemia Enhances Atherosclerosis Regression (ENHANCE), Improved Reduction of Outcomes: Vytorin™ Efficacy International Trial (IMPROVE IT), Simvastatin and Ezetimibe in Aortic Stenosis Study (SEAS), and Study of Heart and Renal Protection (SHARP). These major endpoint trials collectively involve more than 21,000 patients.

3. Conclusions

A wide therapeutic gap exists between target LDL-C levels and LDL-C levels typically achieved in actual clinical practice — a gap that will certainly widen with traditional therapy of single inhibition in light of recent amendments to the NCEP ATP III guidelines. The new aggressive cholesterol treatment goals call for a more advanced therapeutic approach to maximize the cardiovascular benefits associated with lower LDL-C levels. One logical approach is to target both cholesterol production in the liver and absorption in the intestine. By administering ezetimibe/simvastatin as a single tablet or co-administering ezetimibe together with any dose of any statin, we can expect superior LDL-C-lowering efficacy and a substantially greater proportion of patients achieving or getting below LDL-C treatment goals. Treating two sources of cholesterol through Dual Inhibition should therefore be considered as a more advanced therapeutic option for all hypercholesterolemic patients whose LDL-C levels are not appropriately controlled approximately 2–3 months after initiating statin monotherapy. Four large-scale cardiovascular endpoint trials involving more than 21,000 patients are currently underway to determine the impact of Dual Inhibition on patient outcomes.

References

[1] D. Steinberg, J.L. Witztum, Lipoproteins and atherogenesis. Current concepts, JAMA 264 (1990) 3047–3052.

[2] W.P. Castelli, et al., Lipids and risk of coronary heart disease. The Framingham Study, Ann. Epidemiol. 2 (1992) 23–28.

[3] P.W. Wilson, et al., Prevalence of coronary heart disease in the Framingham Offspring Study: role of lipoprotein cholesterols, Am. J. Cardiol. 46 (1980) 649–654.

[4] J. Stamler, D. Wentworth, J.D. Neaton, Is relationship between serum cholesterol and risk of premature death from coronary heart disease continuous and graded? Findings in 356,222 primary screenees of the Multiple Risk Factor Intervention Trial (MRFIT), JAMA 256 (1986) 2823–2828.

[5] The Lipid Research Clinics Coronary Primary Prevention Trial results. I. Reduction in incidence of coronary heart disease, JAMA 251 (1984) 351–364.

[6] J. Shepherd, et al., Prevention of coronary heart disease with pravastatin in men with hypercholesterolemia. West of Scotland Coronary Prevention Study Group, N. Engl. J. Med. 333 (1995) 1301–1307.

[7] R. Collins, et al., Effects of cholesterol-lowering with simvastatin on stroke and other major vascular events in 20536 people with cerebrovascular disease or other high-risk conditions, Lancet 363 (2004) 757–767.

[8] Randomised trial of cholesterol lowering in 4444 patients with coronary heart disease: the Scandinavian Simvastatin Survival Study (4S), Lancet 344 (1994) 1383–1389.

[9] J.R. Downs, et al., Air Force/Texas Coronary Atherosclerosis Prevention Study (AFCAPS/TEXCAPS): additional perspectives on tolerability of long-term treatment with lovastatin, Am. J. Cardiol. 87 (2001) 1074–1079.

[10] V. Manninen, et al., Lipid alterations and decline in the incidence of coronary heart disease in the Helsinki Heart Study, JAMA 260 (1988) 641–651.

[11] M.H. Frick, et al., Helsinki Heart Study: primary-prevention trial with gemfibrozil in middle-aged men with dyslipidemia. Safety of treatment, changes in risk factors, and incidence of coronary heart disease, N. Engl. J. Med. 317 (1987) 1237–1245.

[12] W.G. Goettsch, et al., Statins are less effective in common daily practice among patients with hypercholesterolemia: the REALITY–PHARMO study, Curr. Med. Res. Opin. 20 (2004) 1025–1033.

[13] K.A. Foley, et al., Effectiveness of statin titration on low-density lipoprotein cholesterol goal attainment in patients at high risk of atherogenic events, Am. J. Cardiol. 92 (2003) 79–81.

[14] R.C. Neal, P.H. Jones, Lipid-lowering: can ezetimibe help close the treatment gap? Clevel. Clin. J. Med. 70 (2003) 777–783.

[15] S.M. Grundy, et al., Implications of recent clinical trials for the National Cholesterol Education Program Adult Treatment Panel III Guidelines, J. Am. Coll. Cardiol. 44 (2004) 720–732.

[16] J. Shepherd, Combined lipid lowering drug therapy for the effective treatment of hypercholesterolaemia, Eur. Heart J. 24 (2003) 685–689.

[17] H. Bays, Ezetimibe, Expert Opin. Investig. Drugs 11 (2002) 1587–1604.

[18] S.D. Turley, Cholesterol metabolism and therapeutic targets: rationale for targeting multiple metabolic pathways, Clin. Cardiol. 27 (2004) III16–III21.

[19] S.B. Patel, Ezetimibe: a novel cholesterol-lowering agent that highlights novel physiologic pathways, Curr. Cardiol. Rep. 6 (2004) 439–442.

[20] C.M. Ballantyne, et al., Effect of ezetimibe coadministered with atorvastatin in 628 patients with primary hypercholesterolemia: a prospective, randomized, double-blind trial, Circulation 107 (2003) 2409–2415.

[21] L. Melani, et al., Efficacy and safety of ezetimibe coadministered with pravastatin in patients with primary hypercholesterolemia: a prospective, randomized, double-blind trial, Eur. Heart J. 24 (2003) 717–728.

[22] C. Gagne, et al., Efficacy and safety of ezetimibe added to ongoing statin therapy for treatment of patients with primary hypercholesterolemia, Am. J. Cardiol. 90 (2002) 1084–1091.

[23] B. Kerzner, et al., Efficacy and safety of ezetimibe coadministered with lovastatin in primary hypercholesterolemia, Am. J. Cardiol. 91 (2003) 418–424.

[24] C.M. Ballantyne, et al., Efficacy and safety of ezetimibe co-administered with simvastatin compared with atorvastatin in adults with hypercholesterolemia, Am. J. Cardiol. 93 (2004) 1487–1494.
[25] T. Feldman, et al., Treatment of high-risk patients with ezetimibe plus simvastatin co-administration versus simvastatin alone to attain National Cholesterol Education Program Adult Treatment Panel III low-density lipoprotein cholesterol goals, Am. J. Cardiol. 93 (2004) 1481–1486.
[26] C. Ballantyne, et al., Dose-comparison study of the combination of ezetimibe and simvastatin (Vytorin) versus atorvastatin in patients with hypercholesterolemia. The Vytorin Versus Atorvastatin (VYVA Study), Am. Heart J. 149 (2005) 464–473.
[27] R.P. Cook, Cholesterol. Distribution of sterols in organisms and in tissues, in: R.P. Cook (Ed.), Cholesterol. Chemistry, Biochemistry, and Pathology, Academic Press, Inc., New York, 1958, pp. 145–180.
[28] D.R. Illingworth, P.B. Duell, W.E. Connor, Disorders of lipid metabolism, in: P. Felig, J.D. Baxter, L.A. Frohman (Eds.), Endocrinology and Metabolism, McGraw-Hill, New York, 1995, pp. 1315–1403.
[29] J.M. Dietschy, S.D. Turley, D.K. Spady, Role of liver in the maintenance of cholesterol and low density lipoprotein homeostasis in different animal species, including humans, J. Lipid Res. 34 (1993) 1637–1659.
[30] S.D. Turley, J.M. Dietschy, Sterol absorption by the small intestine, Curr. Opin. Lipidol. 14 (2003) 233–240.
[31] T. Sudhop, D. Lutjohann, K. von Bergmann, Sterol transporters: targets of natural sterols and new lipid lowering drugs, Pharmacol. Ther. 105 (2005) 333–341.
[32] W. Kramer, et al., Aminopeptidase N (CD13) is a molecular target of the cholesterol absorption inhibitor ezetimibe in the enterocyte brush border membrane, J. Biol. Chem. 280 (2005) 1306–1320.
[33] E.J. Smart, R.A. De Rose, S.A. Farber, Annexin 2-caveolin 1 complex is a target of ezetimibe and regulates intestinal cholesterol transport, Proc. Natl. Acad. Sci. U. S. A. 101 (2004) 3450–3455.
[34] M.W. Huff, Dietary cholesterol, cholesterol absorption, postprandial lipemia and atherosclerosis, Can. J. Clin. Pharmacol. 10 (Suppl A) (2003) 26A–32A.
[35] J. Shepherd, Lipids in health and disease, Biochem. Soc. Trans. 32 (2004) 1051–1056.
[36] R.H. Knopp, Drug treatment of lipid disorders, N. Engl. J. Med. 341 (1999) 498–511.
[37] G. Steiner, The need for a different cholesterol lowering drug, Can. J. Clin. Pharmacol. 10 (Suppl A) (2003) 4A–6A.
[38] M. Van Heek, et al., Comparison of the activity and disposition of the novel cholesterol absorption inhibitor, SCH58235, and its glucuronide, SCH60663, Br. J. Pharmacol. 129 (2000) 1748–1754.
[39] M.A. Lavoie, Ezetimibe and cholesterol absorption, Can. J. Clin. Pharmacol. 10 (Suppl A) (2003) 7A–12A.
[40] S.W. Altmann, et al., Niemann–Pick C1 Like 1 protein is critical for intestinal cholesterol absorption, Science 303 (2004) 1201–1204.
[41] U. Seedorf, et al., Cholesterol absorption inhibitor Ezetimibe blocks uptake of oxidized LDL in human macrophages, Biochem. Biophys. Res. Commun. 320 (2004) 1337–1341.
[42] S.E. Nissen, et al., Effect of intensive compared with moderate lipid-lowering therapy on progression of coronary atherosclerosis: a randomized controlled trial, JAMA 291 (2004) 1071–1080.
[43] T. Pearson, et al., Ezetimibe added to statin therapy reduces LDL-C and improves goal attainment in patients with hypercholesterolemia (abstract), American College of Cardiology 53rd Annual Meeting, New Orleans, March 7–10, 2004.
[44] C. Gagne, et al., Efficacy and safety of ezetimibe added to ongoing statin therapy for treatment of patients with primary hypercholesterolemia, Am. J. Cardiol. 90 (2002) 1084–1091.
[45] A.L. Catapano, et al., Lipid-altering efficacy on the ezetimibe/simvastatin single tablet versus rosuvastatin in hypercholesterolemic patients, Curr. Med. Res. Opin. 22 (10) (2006) 2041–2053.

ELSEVIER

International Congress Series 1303 (2007) 129–137

www.ics-elsevier.com

LIFE (losartan intervention for endpoint reduction in hypertension) study and its substudies

Claudio Borghi [a,*], Sibel Ertek [b]

[a] *Dipartimento di Medicina Clinica e Biotecnologia Applicata "D. Campanacci", Università degli Studi di Bologna, Policlinico S. Orsola Via Massarenti 9, 40138 Bologna, Italia*
[b] *Ankara Guven Hospital, Internal Medicine Department, Ankara, Turkey*

Abstract. Hypertension is one of the most important causes of mortality and morbidity in modern world. Its treatment with renin–angiotensin system blockade provides beneficial effects especially in special patient groups. The LIFE (losartan intervention for endpoint reduction in hypertension) study analysed the differences between an angiotensin receptor blocker (losartan) and a beta-blocker (atenolol) antihypertensive treatments in patients with hypertension and left ventricular hypertrophy. Despite similar blood pressure reductions, losartan showed beneficial effects in primary endpoints, and also new-onset diabetes, stroke, albuminuria, left ventricular hypertrophy regression and in atrial fibrillation. Although there are some restrictions on the study, the results show the beneficial effects of angiotensin receptor blockers in hypertensive patients with high risk, with probably mechanisms other than blood pressure reduction.

Keywords: Hypertension; Left ventricular hypertrophy; Losartan; Atenolol

1. Introduction

Hypertension is one of the most important causes of mortality and morbidity all around the world, but only 53% of hypertensive patients with medical treatment achieved the blood pressure levels recommended by the seventh report of the Joint National Committee on prevention, detection, evaluation and treatment of high blood pressure (JNC VII) [1,2]. This may account for significantly higher rates of hypertension-related cardiovascular complications in this patient group.

* Corresponding author. Tel.: +39 051 6363243; fax: +39 051 391320.
E-mail address: claudio.borghi@unibo.it (C. Borghi).

0531-5131/
doi:10.1016/j.ics.2007.03.014

Recent data showed the role of renin–angiotensin system (RAS), and mainly angiotensin II, in hypertension and atherosclerosis [3–9]. And blockade of RAS provides target organ protection in selected patient groups [10–12].

Among all classes of antihypertensive drugs, angiotensin receptor antagonists theoretically provide more complete blockade of RAS at angiotensin receptor level, and they have better side-effect profiles compared with other RAS blocking antihypertensive drugs [13,14].

The losartan intervention for endpoint reduction in hypertension (LIFE) study was started in the early 1990s and at that time there were diuretics and β-blockers as a proven effective treatment for essential hypertension and losartan was compared with atenolol [15].

2. LIFE (losartan intervention for endpoint reduction in hypertension) study

Losartan was the first of a new class of antihypertensive agents blocking angiotensin II at the type 1 receptor level. Angiotensin II is associated with the development of left ventricular hypertrophy that is strong independent indicator of risk of cardiovascular morbidity and death [16]. Thus, blocking angiotensin II could be especially effective in reversing left ventricular hypertrophy. Atenolol was chosen because it was recognised as a first-line treatment for hypertension with similar antihypertensive efficacy to losartan and benefits for secondary cardiovascular protection [17–19]. The major hypothesis of LIFE study is that in patients with essential hypertension and left ventricular hypertrophy, losartan will reduce the incidence of cardiovascular morbidity and mortality to a greater extent than the β-blocker atenolol, possibly through a greater effect on the regression of left ventricular hypertrophy [20]. LIFE is an investigator-initiated, multicenter, double-blind, randomised, prospective, active-controlled parallel group trial in patients with hypertension and left ventricular hypertrophy [20]. The primary endpoint was cardiovascular morbidity and death, a composite endpoint of cardiovascular death, myocardial infarction, and stroke. Other outcome measures were total mortality, angina pectoris or heart failure requiring admission to hospital, coronary or peripheral revascularisation procedures, resuscitated cardiac arrest, and new-onset diabetes mellitus [20]. Men and women between 55 and 80 years of age with previously untreated or treated essential hypertension, with systolic blood pressure of 160 to 200 mm Hg, diastolic blood pressure of 95 to 110 mm Hg, and electrocardiographically documented left ventricular hypertension were included [21]. The patients enrolled from June 1995 to May 1997 in 945 centers. Data of 9193 patients were available for final analyses. Patients were followed for at least 4 years with regular visits and increases in drug doses and addition of hydrochlorothiazide for both drug groups, to reach target blood pressure of less than 140/90 mm Hg (Figs. 1, 2).

Primary endpoints occurred in 1096 patients in 44,119 patient years of follow-up [20]. Target blood pressures were achieved in 49% in losartan and 46% in atenolol groups for systolic blood pressure, in 89% and 89% for diastolic blood pressures, and in 48% and 45% for both. For the primary endpoint, the overall 13.0% relative risk reduction on losartan was seen ($p=0.021$). On individual endpoints, for stroke outcome was highly in favour of losartan, with 24.9% relative risk reduction compared with atenolol ($p=0.001$). Among other prespecified endpoints, the incidence of new-onset diabetes was 25% lower in losartan group. Discontinuation as a result of adverse events was significantly less common in losartan than atenolol patients (for all causes $p<0.0001$, for drug-related causes $p=0.0001$).

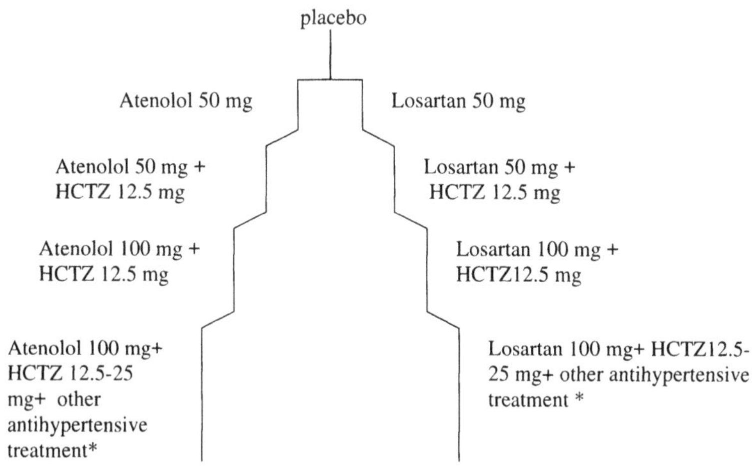

Fig. 1. Titration schedule. *Addition of angiotensin converting enzyme inhibitors, angiotensin II type 1 receptor antagonists, or beta blockers prohibited.

Left ventricular mass was measured at baseline and at the end of the study with two criteria, the Cornell voltage duration product and the Sokolow-Lyon voltage.

A greater reduction of left ventricular mass was attained with losartan than with atenolol, which was independent of blood pressure reduction. This effect may result from a more complete protection against angiotensin II which is myocardial growth factor and independent risk factor for cardiovascular disease [22] with losartan.

Reduction in stroke with losartan is important, because protective effect of ACE (angiotensin-converting enzyme) inhibition was also suggested in HOPE trial, beyond their blood pressure reducing effect [23]. Moreover, left ventricular hypertrophy is a blood-pressure-independent predictor for cardiovascular events [24].

Lower rate of new-onset diabetes is also in concordance with other studies of ACE inhibitors [23,25] and may be related with the effect of this group of drugs on insulin resistance.

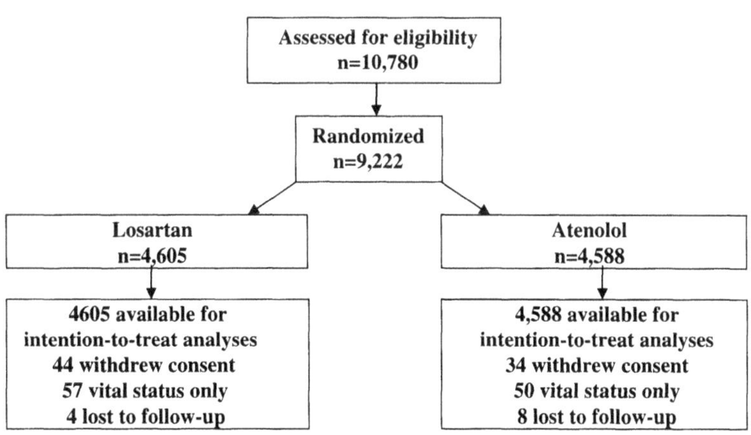

Fig. 2. LIFE study design.

The similar incidences of myocardial infarction with both drugs show the comparable beneficial effects of losartan on myocardium, because β-blockers have proven cardio-protective properties.

The lower rate of adverse effects with losartan may also contribute better patient compliance, which is one of the important problems in hypertensive patient treatment.

When diabetic subgroup of patients have been evaluated separately in LIFE study, among 9193 patients of the study, 13% ($n = 1195$) were diabetic (most likely of type 2 diabetes mellitus) [26]. Losartan was more effective than atenolol in reducing cardiovascular mortality and morbidity as well as mortality from all causes in patients with hypertension, diabetes and left ventricular hypertrophy. In the non-diabetic patients, almost 15% reduction of the primary outcome was mostly driven by the 24% reduction of stroke, but in the subgroup of patients with diabetes, the 24% reduction in primary endpoint was linked to the reduction of cardiovascular and total mortality. Also in diabetic group of patients, losartan was more effective in reversing left ventricular hypertrophy (by both electrocardiographic criteria $p < 0.0001$).

In 8206 patients of LIFE study, changes in albuminuria were evaluated during 4.8 years of antihypertensive treatment and baseline and annual measurements of urinary albumin/creatinine ratio (UACR) was measured [27]. According to median baseline value and median year 1 UACR the patient population was divided to groups and similar significant, stepwise increases were observed for the components of the primary composite endpoint (cardiovascular mortality, stroke and myocardial infarction) which was not explained by in-treatment levels of blood pressure. Thus, these data show that the monitoring of albuminuria is an important part of antihypertensive treatment. In this patient group, the decrease of albuminuria was significantly greater with losartan versus atenolol throughout the study (a decrease from baseline to year 2 of 33% losartan versus 25% atenolol) [28]. The benefits of losartan versus atenolol for the primary composite endpoints and for stroke tended to be more pronounced among the patients above the median value of baseline albuminuria. The decrease in albuminuria was significantly greater with losartan versus atenolol throughout the study (a decrease from baseline to year 2 of 33% losartan versus 25% atenolol). Benefits of losartan seem to be more prominent in patients with the highest levels of baseline UACR, although treatment of albuminuria was only significant for total mortality [29].

In one echocardiographic substudy of LIFE study, left atrial size in patients with left ventricular hypertrophy was evaluated [30]. Left atrial size in these patients was influenced by gender, age, obesity, systolic blood pressure, and left ventricular geometry, independent of left ventricular mass and presence of atrial fibrillation or mitral regurgitation. In another echocardiographically evaluation of LIFE data, in patients with essential hypertension and baseline electrocardiographic left ventricular hypertrophy, lower left ventricular mass during antihypertensive treatment was found to be associated with lower rates of clinical endpoints, additional to effects of blood pressure lowering and treatment modality [31].

3. RAS blockers on treatment or prevention of atrial fibrillation

Animal studies and meta-analyses of data about previous studies show that the treatment with ACEI or ARBs decrease atrial fibrosis, prevent shortening of atrial effective refractory period, prevent atrial structural changes to activate continuation of atrial fibrillation and decrease recurrence [32–41]. AF is associated with increased cardiovascular risk, and the incidence of AF is increased in patients with uncontrolled hypertension [42–44]. Antihypertensive treatment reduces new-onset AF, it is not clear whether there is difference between different groups of these drugs. In the study of Pedersen et al., in patients after acute myocardial infarction, RAS blockade reduces new-onset AF and helps to maintain sinus rhythm [45].

LIFE study data were evaluated to determine whether selective angiotensin II receptor type 1 blockade with losartan was more effective than beta-blockade with atenolol in reducing new-onset AF and associated cardiovascular events in hypertensive patients with electrocardiographic left ventricular hypertrophy. Among 9193 patients of the study, after exclusion of those with AF history or by Minnesota coding of the baseline electrocardiography, 8851 patients were evaluated. New-onset AF occurred in 150 losartan, and 221 atenolol-treated patients (HR=0.67, 95% CI to 0.55 to 0.83, $p<0.001$). And patients taking losartan tended to stay in sinus rhythm longer from the baseline than those taking atenolol (1809±225 versus 1709±254 days from baseline, $p=0.057$).

Although patients of two groups have similar baseline characteristics, losartan-treated patients with new-onset AF had a 40% lower rate of subsequent composite events compared with atenolol-treated patients ($n=31$ versus $n=51$, HR=0.60, 95% CI 0.38 to 0.94, $p=0.03$). Also they have fewer subsequent strokes ($n=19$ versus $n=38$, HR=0.49, 95% CI 0.29 to 0.86, $p=0.01$) fewer myocardial infarctions ($n=9$ versus 16, HR=0.60, 95% CI 0.25 to 1.27, $p=0.16$) and no difference in cardiovascular mortality. In contrast atenolol-treated patients had fewer hospitalisations for heart failure ($n=20$ versus 30, HR=0.43, 95% CI 0.25 to 0.76, $p=0.004$) and a trend toward fewer sudden cardiac deaths ($n=2$ versus 6, HR=0.22, 95% CI 0.05 to 1.10, $p=0.07$). In multivariate prediction models, age (9% higher rate with each year), male gender (56% increase compared to women), systolic blood pressure (6% increase per 10 mm Hg) and electrocardiographically evident left ventricular hypertrophy by Cornell product (4% increase per 100 mV ms) were found and randomisation to losartan was associated with a 33% lower rate of new-onset AF, independent of other risk factors ($p<0.001$) and 51% lower rate of subsequent stroke [46]. In this study losartan reduced the rate of new-onset AF by 33% compared to atenolol with similar blood pressure reduction. This was interesting because beta-blockade is a first-line treatment to prevent AF and it is preferred for the rate control in established AF.

One explanation for the benefit of losartan in new-onset AF in hypertensive patients with left ventricular hypertrophy could be the effects of losartan on regression of atrial and ventricular hypertrophy. LIFE data show that sustained left ventricular hypertrophy is an important predictor of new-onset AF. In LIFE echocardiography substudy it was shown that patients with left ventricular hypertrophy also exhibit increased left atrial size, which has been associated with increased stroke risk in normotensive and hypertensive adults [47–49].

The greater regression of electrocardiographic and echocardiographic left ventricular hypertrophy may be because of greater reduction of left atrial overload and dilatation, thereby reducing stimuli to new-onset AF. But still more experimental data are needed to establish the role of RAS inhibition on cardiac remodelling and AF prevention.

4. Stroke reduction with losartan in hypertensive adults with cardiac hypertrophy

In LIFE study group of patients, with similar blood pressure reductions, 24.9% relative risk reduction with losartan compared with atenolol ($p=0.001$) was achieved (20). Systolic blood pressure <140 mm Hg was achieved in 50% of losartan-treated and 47% of atenolol-treated patients, whereas diastolic blood pressure <90 mm Hg was achieved by 87% of losartan-treated and 89% of atenolol-treated patients. First stokes included 395 (73.0%) ischemic atherothrombotic, 81 (15.0%) ischemic embolic, 55 (10.2%) hemorrhagic, and 10 (1.8%) other events. Among these events, 76 (14.0%) were fatal. Atrial fibrillation at baseline or during the study occurred in 55% of patients with embolic stroke. Recurrent stroke supervened in 72 (13.3%) patients during follow-up. The statistically significant benefits of losartan-based versus atenolol-based therapy in reducing stroke risk extended to ischemic stroke and its major category, atherothrombotic stroke, as well as the fatal stroke [50].

RAS antagonism may lead to cerebral protection beyond its antihypertensive effects [51]. Moreover studies in a model of acute stroke induced by carotid ligation suggest that AT2 receptor stimulation may mediate cerebrovascular anti-ischemic effects [52]. Another additional mechanism that may contribute to the cerebrovascular benefits of losartan is enhanced regression of left ventricular hypertrophy which is an independent risk factor for stroke [53]. In LIFE study group, there were composite endpoints ($n=31$ versus 51, hazard ratio$n=0.60$, 95% CI 0.38 to 0.94, $p=0.03$) and strokes ($n=19$ versus 38, hazard ratio $=0.49$, 95% CI 0.29 to 0.86, $p=0.01$) in patients who developed new-onset AF in the losartan compared to atenolol treatment arm of the study. New-onset AF occurred in 150 patients randomised to losartan versus 221 to atenolol (6.8 versus 10.1 per 1000 person-years; relative risk 0.67, 95% CI 0.55 to 0.83, $p<0.001$) despite similar blood pressure reduction [46].

5. New-onset diabetes

Diabetes mellitus is a disease considered on of the main threats to human health and its prevention is necessary to decrease its undesirable micro- and macrovascular effects [54]. Effects of antihypertensive drugs in the LIFE study, to reduce the risk of new-onset diabetes were evaluated [55]. At baseline, 7998 of patients did not have diabetes mellitus, 562 patients developed diabetes during the study. The new-onset diabetes mellitus occurred in 242 patients with losartan treatment, and 320 patients with atenolol treatment (relative risk $=0.75$, 95% CI, 0.63 to 0.88, $p<0.001$). To identify most important factors to develop diabetes multivariate prediction models were used and it is found that new-onset diabetes could be strongly predicted by baseline serum glucose concentration (non-fasting), body mass index, serum high density lipoprotein cholesterol levels, systolic blood pressure and history of prior use of antihypertensive drugs. Independent of these risk factors, fewer patients with left ventricular hypertrophy developed diabetes mellitus when they are being treated with losartan, compared to atenolol [55].

6. Conclusion

Despite some limitations of the study such as less number of patients from black population, that generally exhibit salt-sensitive, low-renin hypertension, the results of the LIFE study and its substudies can be attributable to the general population of high-risk hypertensive patients. Comparison of beta-blocker atenolol with angiotensin receptor antagonist losartan yielded similar blood pressure decreasing effects and also similar results regarding primary endpoints of the study. This is important because the beta blockers were proved to be first choice drugs for many cardiovascular indications. In the LIFE study, rates of myocardial infarction and hospitalisation for angina pectoris were similar in both drug groups. Especially result about atrial fibrillation opens promising area of investigation about role of RAS blockade in anti-arrhythmic therapy. Prevention of new-onset diabetes with losartan provides the elimination of a new major cardiovascular risk factor in this high-risk patient group. Decreased rates of stroke mean decreased rate of long-term disability and mortality worldwide. In the LIFE study, importance of left ventricular hypertrophy and albuminuria in hypertensive patient follow-up was also discussed. Therefore, this study demonstrated that losartan is more effective than atenolol in the treatment of high-risk hypertensive patients and LIFE study suggests the possibility of some beneficial effects of mechanisms other than blood pressure control by RAS blockade with losartan.

References

[1] I. Hajjar, T. Kotchen, Trends in the prevalence, awareness, treatment, and control of hypertension in the United States, 1988–2000, J. Am. Med. Assoc. 290 (2003) 199–206.
[2] JNC 7 writing committee, The Seventh Report of the Joint National Committee on Prevention, Detection, Evaluation, and Treatment of High Blood Pressure: the JNC 7 report, J. Am. Med. Assoc. 289 (2003) 2560–2572.
[3] H. Rakugi, et al., Induction of angiotensin converting enzyme in the neointima after vascular injury: possible role in restenosis, J. Clin. Invest. 93 (1994) 339–346.
[4] M. Viswanathan, et al., Baloon angioplasty enhances the expression of angiotensin II AT1 receptors in neointima of rat aorta, J. Clin. Invest. 90 (1992) 1707–1712.
[5] V.J. Dazu, Cell biology and genetics of angiotensin in cardiovascular disease, J. Hypertens. 12 (suppl 4) (1994) S3–S10.
[6] K. Grote, H. Drexler, B. Schieffer, Renin–angiotensin system and atherosclerosis, Nephrol. Dial. Transplant. 19 (2004) 770–773.
[7] S. Wassmann, G. Nickenig, Pathophysiological regulation of the AT 1-receptor and implications for vascular disease, J. Hypertens., Suppl. 24 (2006) S15–S21.
[8] Z.J. Cheng, H. Vapaatalo, E. Mervaala, Angiotensin II and vascular inflammation, Med. Sci. Monit. 11 (2005) RA194–RA205.
[9] K.J. Scheidegger, S. Butler, J.L. Witztum, Angiotensin II increases macrophage-mediated modification of low density lipoprotein via a lipoxygenase-dependent pathway, J. Biol. Chem. 272 (1997) 21609–21615.
[10] The Heart Outcomes Prevention Evaluation Study Investigators, Effects of angiotensin-converting enzyme inhibitor, ramipril on cardiovascular events in high risk patients, N. Eng. J. Med. 342 (2000) 145–153.
[11] D. De Zeeuw, et al., Renoprotective effects of rennin–angitensin system inhibitors, Lancet 367 (2006) 899–900.
[12] S.G. Chyrsant, G.S. Chyrsant, The pleiotrophic effects of angiotensin receptor blockers, J. Clin. Hypertens. (Greenwich) 8 (2006) 261–268.
[13] M.A. Weber, Comparison of type 1 angiotensin II receptor blockers and angiotensin converting enzyme inhibitors in the treatment of hypertension, J. Hypertens. 15 (1997) S31–S36 (Suppl).
[14] W.J. Elliot, Therapeutic trials comparing angiotensin converting enzyme inhibitors and angiotensin II receptor blockers, Curr. Hypertens. Rep. 2 (2000) 402–411.
[15] B. Dahlöf, et al., The losartan intervention for endpoint reduction (LIFE) in hypertension study: rationale, design, and methods, Am. J. Hypertens. 10 (1997) 705–713.
[16] S.E. Kjeldsen, et al., Mechanism of angiotensin II type 1 receptor blocker action in the regression of left ventricular hypertrophy, J. Clin. Hypertens. (Greenwich) 8 (2006) 487–492.
[17] B. Dahlöf, et al., Efficacy and tolerability of losartan potassium and atenolol in patients with mild to moderate essential hypertension, Am. J. Hypertens. 8 (1995) 578–583.
[18] L. Hasson, et al., Randomised trial of old and new antihypertensive drugs in elderly patients: cardiovascular mortality and morbidity the Swedish Trial in Old Patients with Hypertension-2 study, Lancet 354 (1999) 1751–1756.

[19] First International Study of Infarct Survival Collaborative Group, Randomised trial of intravenous atenolol among 16027 cases of suspected acute myocardial infarction: ISIS-1, Lancet 2 (1986) 57–66.
[20] B. Dahlöf, et al., Cardiovascular morbidity and mortality in the losartan intervention for endpoint reduction in hypertension study (LIFE): a randomised trial against atenolol, Lancet 359 (2002) 995–1003.
[21] B. Dahlöf, et al., Characteristics of 9194 patients with left ventricular hypertrophy: the LIFE study. Losartan intervention for endpoint reductions in hypertension, Hypertension 32 (1998) 989–997.
[22] M. Nemer, Mechanisms of angiotensin II. Dependent progression to heart failure, Novartis Found. Symp. 274 (2006) 58–68.
[23] S. Yusuf, et al., Effects of an angiotensin-converting enzyme inhibitor, ramipril on cardiovascular events in high risk patients: the Heart Outcomes Prevention Evaluation study investigators, N. Engl. J. Med. 342 (2000) 145–153.
[24] P. Verdecchia, et al., Left ventricular hypertrophy as an independent predictor of acute cerebrovascular events in essential hypertension, Circulation 104 (2001) 2039–2044.
[25] L. Hasson, et al., Effect of angiotensin-converting-enzyme-inhibition compared with conventional therapy on cardiovascular morbidity and mortality in hypertension: the Captopril Prevention Project (CAPP) randomised trial, Lancet 353 (1999) 611–616.
[26] L.H. Lindholm, et al., Cardiovascular morbidity and mortality in patients with diabetes in the losartan intervention for endpoint reduction in hypertension study (LIFE): a randomised trial against atenolol, Lancet 359 (2002) 1004–1010.
[27] H. Ibsen, et al., Reduction in albuminuria translates to reduction in cardiovascular events in hypertensive patients: losartan intervention for endpoint reduction in hypertension study, Hypertension 45 (2005) 181–182.
[28] H. Ibsen, et al., Does albuminuria predict cardiovascular outcome on treatment with losartan versus atenolol in hypertension with left ventricular hypertrophy? A LIFE substudy, J. Hypertens. 22 (2004) 1679–1681.
[29] H. Ibsen, et al., Does albuminuria predict cardiovascular outcomes on treatment with losartan versus atenolol in patients with diabetes, hypertension, and left ventricular hypertrophy? The LIFE study, Diabetes Care 29 (2006) 595–600.
[30] E. Gerdts, et al., Correlates of left atrial size in hypertensive patients with left ventricular hypertrophy: the LIFE study, Hypertension 39 (2002) 739–743.
[31] R.B. Deverux, et al., Prognostic significance of left ventricular mass change during treatment of hypertension, JAMA 292 (2004) 2396–2398.
[32] D. Li, et al., Effects of angiotensin-converting enzyme inhibition on the development of the atrial fibrillation substrate in dogs with ventricular tachypacing-induced congestive heart failure, Circulation 104 (2001) 2608–2614.
[33] Y. Shi, Enalapril effects on atrial remodelling and atrial fibrillation in experimental congestive heart failure, Cardiovasc. Res. 54 (2002) 456–461.
[34] K. Kumagai, et al., Effect of angiotensin II type 1 receptor antagonist on electrical and structural remodelling in atrial fibrillation, J. Am. Coll. Cardiol. 41 (2003) 2197–2204.
[35] H. Nakashima, et al., Angiotensin II antagonist prevents electrical remodelling in atrial fibrillation, Circulation 101 (2000) 2612–2617.
[36] J.S. Kalus, C.I. Coleman, M. White, The impact of suppressing the rennin-angiotensin system on atrial fibrillation, J. Clin. Pharmacol. 46 (2006) 21–28.
[37] A.H. Madrid, et al., The role of angiotensin receptor blockers and/or angiotensin converting enzyme inhibitors in the prevention of atrial fibrillation in patients with cardiovascular diseases: meta-analysis of randomized controlled clinical trials, Pacing Clin. Electrophysiol. 27 (2004) 1405–1410.
[38] J.S. Healey, et al., Prevention of atrial fibrillation with angiotensin-converting enzyme inhibitors and angiotensin receptor blockers: a meta-analysis, J. Am. Coll. Cardiol. 45 (2005) 1832–1839.
[39] A.H. Madrid, et al., Prevention of recurrence in patients with lone atrial fibrillation. The dose-dependent effect of angiotensin II receptor blockers, J. Renin Angiotensin Aldosterone Syst. 5 (2004) 114–120.
[40] A.H. Madrid, et al., Use of irbesartan to maintain sinus rhythm in patients with long-lasting persistent atrial fibrillation: a prospective and randomized study, Circulation 106 (2002) 331–336.
[41] K.C. Ueng, et al., Use of enalapril to facilitate sinus rhythm maintenance after external cardioversion of long-standing persistent atrial fibrillation: results of a prospective and controlled study, Eur. Heart J. 24 (2003) 2090–2098.

[42] S. Stewart, et al., A population-based study of the long-term risks associated with atrial fibrillation. 20 year follow-up of the Renfrew/Paisley Study, Am. J. Med. 113 (2002) 359–364.
[43] H. Vidaillet, et al., A population-based study of mortality among patients with atrial fibrillation or flutter, Am. J. Med. 113 (2002) 365–367.
[44] T.S. Tsang, et al., The prevalence of atrial fibrillation in incident stroke cases and matched population controls in Rochester, Minnesota: changes over three decades, Am. J. Coll. Cardiol. 42 (2003) 93–100.
[45] O.D. Pedersen, et al., Trandolapril reduces the incidence of atrial fibrillation after acute myocardial infarction in patients with left ventricular dysfunction, Circulation 100 (1999) 376–380.
[46] K. Watchell, et al., Angiotensin II receptor blockade reduces new-onset atrial fibrillation and subsequent stroke compared to atenolol. The losartan intervention for endpoint reduction in hypertension (LIFE) study, J. Am. Coll. Cardiol. 45 (2005) 712–719.
[47] E. Gerdts, et al., Correlates of left atrial size in hypertensive patients with left ventricular hypertrophy: the losartan intervention for endpoint reduction in hypertension (LIFE) study, Hypertension 39 (2002) 739–743.
[48] E.J. Benjamin, et al., Left atrial size and the risk of stroke and death.The Framingham Heart study, Circulation 92 (1995) 835–841.
[49] J.S. Gottdiener, et al., Effect of single drug therapy on reduction of left atrial size in mild to moderate hypertension: comparison of six antihypertensive agents, Circulation 98 (1998) 140–148.
[50] J.R. Kizer, et al., Stroke reduction in hypertensive adults with cardiac hypertrophy randomised to losartan versus atenolol: the losartan intervention for endpoint reduction in hypertension study, Hypertension 45 (2005) 46–52.
[51] C.T. Stier, et al., Stroke prevention by losartan in stroke prone spontaneously hypertensive rats, J. Hypertens. 11 (suppl. 3) (1993) S37–S42.
[52] J.M. Achard, et al., Protection against ischemia: a physiological function of the renin–angiotensin system, Biochem. Pharmacol. 62 (2001) 261–271.
[53] P. Verdecchia, et al., Left ventricular hypertrophy as an independent predictor of acute cerebrovascular events in essential hypertension, Circulation 104 (2001) 2039–2044.
[54] P. Zimmet, K.G. Alberti, J. Shaw, Global and societal implications of the diabetic epidemic, Nature 414 (2001) 782–787.
[55] L.H. Lindholm, et al., Risk of new-onset diabetes in the losartan intervention for endpoint reduction in hypertension study, J. Hypertens. 20 (2002) 1879–1886.

ELSEVIER

International Congress Series 1303 (2007) 138 – 145

www.ics-elsevier.com

When and how to restore β-cell function?

Francesca Pancani *, Roberto Lupi, Roberto Miccoli, Piero Marchetti, Stefano Del Prato

Department of Endocrinology & Metabolism, Section of Diabetes and Metabolic Disease, Cisanello Hospital, Pisa, Italy

Abstract. Diabetes is due to the concomitant presence of insulin resistance and impaired insulin secretion. β-Cell dysfunction begins during the prediabetic period, is progressive and not modified by the used therapy. It seems to be determined also by the genetic pattern, and some variants of *TCF7L2* gene show in recent reports the strongest association with the alteration of both β-cell function and mass. New therapeutic approaches should therefore improve not only the function but also the β-cell mass. To this aim, strict glycemic control, insulin-sensitizers such as thiazolidinediones and incretin mimetic molecules can be used. © 2007 Published by Elsevier B.V.

Keywords: β-Cell function; β-Cell mass; Insulin secretion

1. Introduction

Type 2 diabetes (T2DM) is characterized by the concomitance of two defects: insulin resistance and impaired insulin secretion [1,2]. Insulin resistance is a common defect not only in patients with overt diabetes but also in subjects with impaired glucose tolerance and even in individuals at high risk of developing diabetes [3]. For this reason, insulin resistance has been considered the hallmark of T2DM [1]. However, overt hyperglycemia does not develop until the defect in insulin sensitivity can be compensated by increased insulin secretion. Previous studies have shown that plasma insulin concentrations after an OGTT progressively increase with the elevation of fasting plasma glucose, eventually decreasing upon development of marked fasting hyperglycemia (~ 180 mg/dl). Based on these observations DeFronzo postulated the existence of a "Starling curve" of the pancreas [3].

* Corresponding author.
E-mail address: frapanca@tin.it (F. Pancani).

0531-5131/ © 2007 Published by Elsevier B.V.
doi:10.1016/j.ics.2007.03.029

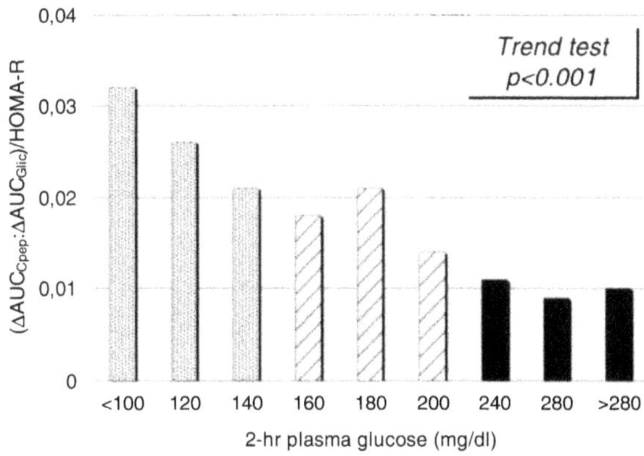

Fig. 1. Insulin secretion (insulinogenic index) corrected insulin action (HOMA-IR) declines across the entire spectrum of glucose tolerance. Of interest is that the drop occurs already within the normal glucose tolerance range. Grey columns = normal glucose tolerance range; cross-hatched columns = impaired glucose tolerance range; filled columns = diabetes.

This view implicates the concept that chronic and progressive demand imposed on the β-cell by insulin resistance, along with intoxication due to high glucose concentration (glucotoxicity), leads to β-cell exhaustion. The same concept implies that the defect in β-cell function is, to some extent, secondary to insulin resistance and altered metabolic milieu.

This view has been challenged by the results of the UKPDS [4]. By using the HOMA-B as a surrogate of β-cell function two main features have been identified: (1) a marked reduction of β-cell function (~ 50%) at the time of diabetes diagnosis, and (2) progressive reduction of β-cell function irrespective of the form of antidiabetic therapy used. Such a reduction was linear to the point that backward extrapolation suggested that β-cell defect can precede by many years the development of overt diabetes. To a similar conclusion has come the Belfast Diet Study [5]. By mathematical modeling of data from subjects with different duration of disease and different degrees of metabolic control, a biphasic course of β-cell function was described [6]. This course is characterized by a first phase (phase A) occurring during the prediabetic period when β-cell function was calculated to a decay rate of ~2% and a second one (phase B), after diabetes diagnosis, when reduction of β-cell function proceeded at faster rate (~ 18% per year).

These observations clearly support the hypothesis that a defect of β-cell function is occurring at much earlier stages than previously suggested. Such a view is in keeping with studies indicating loss of first phase insulin secretion for fasting plasma glucose levels of 110 mg/dl [7] as well as with data indicating marked reduction in the β-cell mass already in individuals with IGT [8]. The data also fit with some recent observations of ours. In a group of subjects with different glucose tolerance, insulin sensitivity was determined as HOMA-insulin resistance (HOMA-IR), while post-OGTT plasma C-peptide concentrations were analyzed with a minimal model for C-peptide kinetics, to estimate β-cell secretory capacity (β-index) [9]. IGT and T2DM subjects had similar impairment of insulin sensitivity, whereas the β-index progressively declined from NGT to IGT and diabetes. We are currently running a study designed to identify physiopathologic and genetic markers for the evolution of IFG/IGT patients toward T2DM: the Genetic and Physiopathologic Evolution of T2DM Study (GENFIEV). Almost 1300 individuals have been recruited all across Italy for an OGTT screening allowing identification of NGT (50%), IFG and/or IGT (35%), and type 2 diabetes (15%). By exploring the insulinogenic index as a function of prevalent insulin sensitivity (HOMA-IR) in the whole population based on 20 mg/dl increment above 100 mg/dl 2-h plasma glucose, a large reduction of β-cell function became apparent even within the range of normal glucose tolerance (Fig. 1).

Such an early impairment in β-cell function can only reflect intrinsic predisposition toward failure, a predisposition most likely based on the genetic profile of each individual.

2. Lots of genes, but little satisfaction

There is no doubt that genetic predisposition plays a major role in diabetes development. Nonetheless, with the exception of rare monogenic forms of diabetes (MODY, neonatal diabetes), the genetic pattern for common T2DM form is extremely heterogeneous and many genes are likely to be simultaneously involved. Among these, there are few variants with a demonstrated link to T2DM susceptibility, as PI2A variant in PPARγ and E23K in KCNJ11 [10,11]. Still, these variants confer limited risk, and cannot offer a clinically useful predictive testing. Much greater expectation has been generated by recent reports on variants of *TCF7L2* gene.

Grant et al., by studying the homogeneous Iceland population, found a strong association between a microsatellite marker (DG10S478) within intron 3 of the *TCF7L2* gene on chromosome 10q25.2 and T2DM. In particular, two SNPs (rs12255372 and rs7903146), in strict linkage disequilibrium with DG10S478, were shown to be highly associated with T2DM. This finding has been confirmed in a Danish and in US cohort [12]. Compared with non-carriers, hetero- and homozygous carriers of minor risk alleles had relative risk for T2DM of 1.45 and 2.41 respectively, translating in a population attributable risk of 21%. Further replication of these findings have been obtained in Dutch and in Finnish cohorts [13], where the minor alleles of both variants were over-represented in T2DM groups. The association holds also for non-Caucasian populations such as Indians [14]. In summary, TCF7L2 appears as the strongest T2DM genetic association so far observed, an association supported by both case control and familial transmission disequilibrium studies. This strong association still requires careful phenotype linkage in order to fully understand which pathophysiologic mechanisms are determined. In a general non-selected population, Cauchi et al. [15] showed the T allele variation at rs7903146 to predict prevalence and incidence of hyperglycemia during a 9-year follow-up. No association was found with insulin sensitivity whereas weak association emerged between risk allele and insulin secretion, estimated as fasting insulin levels and HOMA-B.

In the DPP study, two major involved SNPs have been genotyped in IGT subjects to confirm the association observed in prior cross-sectional studies and elucidate the effect of these variants on insulin secretion and insulin sensitivity. Homozygous for the T allele at rs7903146 and rs12255372 were more likely to have progression to diabetes, and their basal insulin secretion (insulin:glucose ratio and corrected insulin response) was significantly lower than CC and GG homozygotes, respectively. On the other hand insulin sensitivity was not worse in TT homozygotes suggestive for a main link between risk alleles and β-cell function [16]. Frequently sampled IVGTT for assessment of insulin secretion and calculation of the disposition index (DI) have been performed in a non-diabetic population of European and African American women by Munoz et al. [17]. While there was no difference in insulin resistance as a function of TCF7L2 variants, homozygous individuals for the SNP rs12255372 T allele had lower AIR_g. Similar results are shown in non-diabetic individuals after an OGTT: homozygous subjects for the rs7903146 risk allele have a 50% reduction in the insulinogenic index (measure of early insulin response to glucose) and insulin disposition index [18].

Whether the association between TCF7L2 variants and β-cell function reflects direct or indirect effects on the β-cell remains to be defined, as both are a possibility. Modulation of Wnt signal pathway in intestinal L-cells may affect pro-glucagon cleavage and GLP-1 release, influencing indirectly insulin secretion. On the other hand, TCF7L2 is expressed in human pancreas leaving open the possibility that a direct effect may be played at the β-cell level and, possibly, α-cell resulting in modulation of both insulin and glucagon release. This scenario is quite fascinating, given the pancreatic bi-hormonal disturbance that characterizes T2DM. In these patients, indeed, impaired insulin secretion is almost always associated with high circulating plasma levels of glucagon leading to reduced insulin:glucagon ratio [19], a factor that exerts a strict control on hepatic glucose metabolism [20].

3. β-Cell: when function and mass do not team up together

Intriguing enough, a possible role of *TCF7L2* may then be exerted on both β-cell function and survival.

β-Cell mass is regulated by a dynamic process in which expansion and involution (shrinkage) are balanced, in response to insulin demand, for maintenance of glucose homeostasis [21]. Remodeling happens, thanks to death and regeneration [22], and involves genetic, metabolic, and environmental factors. In healthy subject β-cell regeneration is perfectly balanced by reduction via cell death, that results from necrosis and/or apoptosis [23,24]. As demonstrated by Flier, in non-diabetic animals β-cell hyperplasia develops in response to insulin resistance [25]. In their experimental work, they transplanted normal islets under the kidney capsule of normoglycemic insulin-resistant mice with two different models of insulin resistance: lean mice that have a double heterozygous deletion of the insulin receptor and insulin receptor substrate-1 (DH) or the obese, hyperglycemic ob/ob mice. In the grafts transplanted into both hosts, there was a marked increase in β-cell mitotic activity and islet mass that was comparable with that observed in the endogenous pancreas. By contrast, islets of the DH mouse transplanted into normal mice showed reduced mitotic index. These data suggest that insulin resistance can be effectively coped with by a normal β-cell, implying that evolution toward hyperglycemia requires a predisposed β-cell. Through hypertrophy and hyperplasia insulin biosynthesis and release can be increased [21,26]. However, these changes may result in greater susceptibility of the β-cell to apoptotic insult [27]. Butler et al. [8] reported that β-cell mass is reduced by 50% in obese subjects with impaired fasting glucose (IFG) and by 63% in obese patients with T2DM. This reduction was entirely accounted for by increased apoptosis, since regeneration was similar in control and T2DM islets.

4. Therapeutic perspectives

From the brief analysis of the current knowledge on the pathophysiologic role of β-cell function in the development of T2DM two main points arise: (1) β-cell defect is an early one in the natural history of diabetes, and (2) pharmacologic intervention should improve function while preserving, if not increasing, β-cell mass. So far sulphonylureas and glinides have been used to stimulate insulin secretion in T2DM patients. In the UKPDS, treatment with sulphonylureas was not associated with any change in the decay curve of β-cell function, being similar to that observed for metformin, bed-time insulin, or diet [28]. Moreover, these compounds have been claimed to favor apoptosis and therefore loss of β-cell mass [29].

A new therapeutic era has been opened up by the incretin concept. It was realized many years ago that insulin response following oral ingestion of glucose is greater than the one elicited by a similar i.v. glucose load [30]. While this effect may account for up to 60% of postprandial insulin secretion of normal individuals, in patients with T2DM it is quite reduced [31]. The incretin effect depends on the rapid release by the gut of several hormonal factors in response to the ingestion of nutrients. Among these factors, gastrointestinal peptide (GIP) and glucagon-like peptide-1 (GLP-1) play a major role. The latter, in particular, has been shown to stimulate insulin secretion [32], suppress glucagon release [33] and normalize blood glucose levels without causing hypoglycemia [34]. However, native GLP-1 is degraded rapidly [35,36] upon intravenous or subcutaneous administration, and is therefore not feasible for routine therapy. To overcome this major limitation two pharmacological strategies have been pursued: (1) molecules (e.g., exenatide and liraglutide) that mimic the incretin effect of GLP-1 but are resistant to dipeptidyl peptidase-IV (DPP-IV), the enzyme that degrades GLP-1; and (2) molecules that inhibit DPP-IV, thereby enhancing the half-life and incretin effects of GLP-1.

Of the first approach, exenatide [37] is now available for clinical applications. Exenatide (exendin-4) is a 39-amino-acid peptide incretin mimetic that exhibits glucoregulatory activities similar to GLP-1. These actions include glucose-dependent enhancement of insulin secretion, suppression of inappropriately high glucagon secretion, and slowing of gastric emptying. Published results from three large 6-month trials [38–40] performed in patients with T2DM indicate that addition of exenatide to classic oral agents results in an average 1.0% reduction in HbA1c together with moderate though consistent weight loss. The same studies showed that improvement in glycemic control was associated with reduced proinsulin-to-insulin ratio suggesting a beneficial effect on the ß-cell.

Sitagliptin has been recently approved by FDA with vildagliptin, and saxagliptin to follow soon after. A 0.7% placebo-adjusted reduction of HbA1c has been reported with vildagliptin with no significant changes in body weight [41]. Twenty-four-hour plasma insulin profile did not change in absolute terms. However, this occurred in the face of significantly lower plasma glucose concentration suggesting improved β-cell function. Assessment of insulin response to a mixed meal by mathematical model analysis indicates that vildagliptin improves β-cell function in the short (28 days) and long run (52 weeks) [42,43].

In vitro and animal data have demonstrated that GLP-1 increases beta-cell mass by stimulating islet cell neogenesis and by inhibiting apoptosis [44]. An ability to stimulate β-cell replication in vitro followed by upregulated expression of the transcription factor PDX-1 (which is involved in pancreatic development, islet cell function, regulation of insulin gene expression, and the increase of β-cell mass in animal models) has also been ascribed to GLP-1 [45]. Even in older, glucose-intolerant rats, GLP-1 stimulated a reversal of the age-related decline in β-cell function. In the light of these experimental results, specific studies are needed to determine to what extent they can be translated to human diseased conditions.

Though thiazolidinediones (TZDs) were introduced as insulin sensitizing agents, a potential role in preserving and improving β-cell function has been postulated [46]. An improvement of β-cell function (HOMA-B) has been reported in several clinical trials employing TZDs [47–51]. A favourable effect is also supported by improvement of insulin processing as shown by a reduction of the proinsulin to insulin ratio [52,53]. The effect on β-cell function may be mediated via relief of gluco-lipotoxicity, but the possibility exists that PPARγ agonists may exert a direct protection of the pancreatic islets, maybe activating the insulin signaling pathway [54]. Preclinical studies in the Zucker diabetic fatty rat demonstrated that rats administered rosiglitazone prior to the onset of overt diabetes remained normoglycemic [55]. These findings indicate that TZDs have the potential to prevent or reverse the clinical progression to type 2 diabetes, as indicated by the TRIPOD and DREAM study [56,57].

5. Conclusions

In summary, β-cell dysfunction becomes manifest early in the natural history of T2DM and is heralded by initial loss of first phase insulin secretion and reduction of β-cell mass. Insulin resistance, chronic hyperglycemia, increased FFA levels may all contribute in accelerating impairment in the β-cell function. Strict metabolic control, then, may relieve some of the demand and pressure put on the islet function. In conclusion, preservation of β-cell must be addressed at very early stage of the disease. This may require improvement of insulin action to reduce demand on β-cell. Insulin sensitizers, such as TZDs, may have a direct effect on presenving β-cell function and survival. More recent acquisitions, such as incretin mimetic molecules and DPP-IV inhibitors, are an interesting opportunity as they target β-cell in both terms of restoring insulinic response after a meal ingestion as well as potentially preserving β-cell mass.

References

[1] M. Stumvoll, H. Haring, Insulin resistance and insulin sensitizers, Horm. Res. 55 (Suppl 2) (2001) 3–13.
[2] J.L. Leahy, Pathogenesis of type 2 diabetes mellitus, Arch. Med. Res. 36 (2005) 197–209.
[3] M.A. Abdul-Ghani, et al., Insulin secretion and insulin action in subjects with impaired fasting and impaired glucose tolerance: results from the Veterans Administration Genetic Epidemiology Study (VEGAS), Diabetes (2006) 1430–1435.
[4] American Diabetes Association, UK Prospective Diabetes Study 16. Overview of 6 years' therapy of type II diabetes: a progressive disease. UK Prospective Diabetes Study (UKPDS) Group, Diabetes 44 (1995) 1249–1258.
[5] J. Levy, et al., Beta-cell deterioration determines the onset and rate of progression of secondary dietary failure in type 2 diabetes mellitus: the 10-year follow-up of the Belfast Diet Study, Diabet. Med. 15 (1998) 290–296.
[6] A. Bagust, S. Beale, Deteriorating beta-cell function in type 2 diabetes: a long-term model, QJM 96 (2003) 281–288.
[7] S. Del Prato, A. Tiengo, The importance of first phase insulin secretion: implications for the therapy of type 2 diabetes mellitus, Diabetes/Metab. Res. Rev. 17 (2001) 164–174.

[8] A.E. Butler, et al., Beta-cell deficit and increased beta-cell apoptosis in humans with type 2 diabetes, Diabetes 52 (2003) 102–110.
[9] A. Cretti, et al., Assessment of beta-cell function during the oral glucose tolerance test by a minimal model of insulin secretion, Eur. J. Clin. Invest. 31 (2001) 405–416.
[10] D. Altshuler, et al., The common PPARgamma Pro12Ala polymorphism is associated with decreased risk of type 2 diabetes, Nat. Genet. 26 (2000) 76–80.
[11] A.L. Gloyn, et al., Large-scale association studies of variants in genes encoding the pancreatic beta-cell KATP channel subunits Kir6.2 (KCNJ11) and SUR1 (ABCC8) confirm that the KCNJ11 E23K variant is associated with type 2 diabetes, Diabetes 52 (2003) 568–572.
[12] S.F. Grant, et al., Variant of transcription factor 7-like 2 (*TCF7L2*) gene confers risk of type 2 diabetes, Nat. Genet. 38 (2006) 320–323.
[13] L.J. Scott, et al., Association of transcription factor 7-like 2 (TCF7L2) variants with type 2 diabetes in a Finnish sample, Diabetes 55 (2006) 2649–2653.
[14] G.R. Chandak, et al., Common variants in the *TCF7L2* gene are strongly associated with type 2 diabetes mellitus in the Indian population, Diabetologia 50 (2007) 63–67.
[15] S. Cauchi, P. Froguel, et al., TCF7L2 variation predicts hyperglycemia incidence in a French general population: the data from an epidemiological study on the Insulin Resistance Syndrome (DESIR) study, Diabetes 55 (2006) 3189–3192.
[16] J.C. Florez, et al., TCF7L2 polymorphisms and progression to diabetes in the Diabetes Prevention Program, NEJM 355 (2006) 241–250.
[17] Munoz, et al., Polymorphism in the transcription factor 7-like 2 (*TCF7L2*) gene is associated with reduced insulin secretion in nondiabetic women, Diabetes 55 (2006) 3630–3634.
[18] C.M. Damcott, et al., Polymorphisms in the transcription factor 7-like 2 (*TCF7L2*) gene are associated with type 2 diabetes in the Amish: replication and evidence for a role in both insulin secretion and insulin resistance, Diabetes 55 (2006) 2654–2659.
[19] S. Del Prato, P. Marchetti, Beta-and alpha-cell dysfunction in type 2 diabetes, Horm. Metab. Res. 36 (2004) 775–781.
[20] R. Taylor, et al., Direct assessment of liver glycogen storage by 13C nuclear magnetic resonance spectroscopy and regulation of glucose homeostasis after a mixed meal in normal subjects, J. Clin. Invest. 97 (1996) 126–132.
[21] C. Bernard-Kargar, A. Ktorza, Endocrine pancreas plasticity under physiological and pathological conditions, Diabetes 50 (Suppl 1) (2001) S30–S35.
[22] S. Del Prato, et al., β-Cell mass plasticity in type 2 diabetes, Diabetes Obes. Metab. 6 (2004) 319–331.
[23] J. Chandra, et al., Role of apoptosis in pancreatic beta-cell death in diabetes, Diabetes 50 (Suppl 1) (2001) S44–S47.
[24] T. Mandrup-Poulsen, Beta-cell apoptosis: stimuli and signaling, Diabetes 50 (Suppl 1) (2001) S58–S63.
[25] S. Flier, et al., Evidence for a circulating islet cell growth factor in insulin-resistant states, PNAS 98 (2001) 7475–7480.
[26] S. Bonner-Weir, Life and death of the pancreatic β-cells, Trends Endocrinol. Metab. 11 (9) (2000) 375–378.
[27] S. Bonner-Weir, Beta-cell turnover: its assessment and implications, Diabetes 50 (Suppl 1) (2001) S20–S24.
[28] D.R. Matthews, et al., Sulphonylurea failure in non-insulin-dependent diabetic patients over six years. UK Prospective Diabetes Study (UKPDS) Group, Diabet. Med. 15 (4) (1998) 297–303.
[29] K. Maedler, et al., Sulfonylurea induced beta-cell apoptosis in cultured human islets, J. Clin. Endocrinol. Metab. 90 (2005) 501–506.
[30] H. Elrick, et al., Plasma insulin responses to oral and intravenous glucose administration, J. Clin. Endocrinol. Metab. 24 (1964) 1076–1082.
[31] M. Nauck, et al., Reduced incretin effect in type 2 diabetes, Diabetologia 29 (1986) 46–54.
[32] B. Kreymann, et al., Glucagon-like peptide 1 7–36: a physiological incretin in man, Lancet (2) (1987) 1300–1304.
[33] T. Matsuyama, et al., Glucagon-like peptide-1 (7–36 amide): a potent glucagonostatic and insulinotropic hormone, Diabetes Res. Clin. Pract. 5 (1988) 281–284.
[34] M. Nauck, et al., Normalization of fasting hyperglycaemia by exogenous glucagon-like peptide 1 (7–36 amide) in type 2 (non-insulin dependent) diabetic patients, Diabetologia 36 (1993) 741–744.
[35] R. Mentlein, B. Gallwitz, W.E. Schmidt, Dipeptidyl-peptidase IV hydrolyses gastric inhibitory polypeptide, glucagon-like peptide-1(7–36) amide, peptide histidine methionine and is responsible for their degradation in human serum, Eur. J. Biochem. 214 (1993) 829–835.

[36] T.J. Kieffer, C.H. McIntosh, R.A. Pederson, Degradation of glucose-dependent insulinotropic polypeptide and truncated glucagon-like peptide 1 in vitro and in vivo by dipeptidyl peptidase IV, Endocrinology 136 (1995) 3585–3596.
[37] L.L. Want, et al., Exenatide and pramlintide: new therapies for diabetes, Int. J. Clin. Pract. 60 (12) (2006) 1522–1523.
[38] J.B. Buse, et al., Effects of exenatide (exendin-4) on glycemic control over 30 weeks in sulfonylurea-treated patients with type 2 diabetes, Diabetes Care 27 (11) (2004) 2628–2635.
[39] R.A. DeFronzo, et al., Effects of exenatide (exendin-4) on glycemic control and weight over 30 weeks in metformin-treated patients with type 2 diabetes, Diabetes Care 28 (5) (2005) 1092–1100.
[40] D.M. Kendall, et al., Effects of exenatide (exendin-4) on glycemic control over 30 weeks in patients with type 2 diabetes treated with metformin and a sulfonylurea, Diabetes Care 28 (5) (2005) 1083–1091.
[41] R.E. Pratley, et al., Twelve-week monotherapy with the DPP-4 inhibitor vildagliptin improves glycemic control in subjects with type 2 diabetes, Horm. Metab. Res. 38 (6) (2006) 423–428.
[42] A. Mari, et al., Vildagliptin, a dipeptidyl peptidase-IV inhibitor, improves model-assessed ß-cell function in patients with type 2 diabetes, J. Clin. Endocrinol. Metab. 90 (8) (2005) 4888–4894.
[43] B. Ahren, et al., Improved meal-related beta-cell function and insulin sensitivity by the dipeptidyl peptidase-IV inhibitor vildagliptin in metformin-treated patients with type 2 diabetes over 1 year, Diabetes Care 28 (8) (2005) 1936–1940.
[44] Q. Wang, et al., Glucagon-like peptide-1 regulates proliferation and apoptosis via activation of protein kinase B in pancreatic INS-1 beta cells, Diabetologia 47 (3) (2004) 478–487.
[45] L. Bai, G. Meredith, B.E. Tuch, Glucagon-like peptide-1 enhances production of insulin in insulin-producing cells derived from mouse embryonic stem cells, J. Endocrinol. 186 (2) (2005) 343–352.
[46] L.A. Leiter, Beta-cell preservation: a potential role for thiazolidinediones to improve clinical care in type 2 diabetes, Diabet. Med. 22 (2005) 963–972.
[47] H.E. Lebovitz, et al., Rosiglitazone monotherapy is effective in patients with type 2 diabetes, J. Clin. Endocrinol. Metab. 86 (2001) 280–288.
[48] B.H. Wolffenbuttel, et al., Addition of low-dose rosiglitazone to sulphonylurea therapy improves glycaemic control in type 2 diabetic patients, Diabet. Med. 17 (2000) 40–47.
[49] D. Einhorn, et al., Pioglitazone hydrochloride in combination with metformin in the treatment of type 2 diabetes mellitus: a randomized, placebo-controlled study. The Pioglitazone 027 Study Group, Clin. Ther. 22 (2000) 1395–1409.
[50] T.A. Jones, et al., Addition of rosiglitazone to metformin is effective in obese, insulin-resistant patients with type 2 diabetes, Diabetes Obes. Metab. 5 (2003) 163–170.
[51] Y. Miyazaki, et al., Improved glycemic control and enhanced insulin sensitivity in type 2 diabetic subjects treated with pioglitazone, Diabetes Care 24 (2001) 710–719.
[52] L.E. Porter, et al., Rosiglitazone reduces proinsulin/insulin ratio and improves b-cell function in type 2 diabetes, Diabetologia 43 (Suppl. 1) (2000) A192.
[53] T.M. Wallace, J.C. Levy, D.R. Matthews, An increase in insulin sensitivity and basal β-cell function in diabetic subjects treated with pioglitazone in a placebo-controlled randomized study, Diabet. Med. 21 (2004) 568–576.
[54] R. Lupi, et al. Personal data.
[55] D.T. Finegood, B. Topp, β-Cell deterioration—prospects for reversal or prevention, Diabetes Obes. Metab. 3 (2001) S20–S27.
[56] S.P. Azen, et al., TRIPOD (TRoglitazone In the Prevention Of Diabetes): a randomized, placebo-controlled trial of troglitazone in women with prior gestational diabetes mellitus, Control Clin. Trials 19 (1998) 217–231.
[57] DREAM (Diabetes Reduction Assessment with ramipril and rosiglitazone Medication) Trial Investigators: Gerstein HC, Yusuf S, Bosch J, Pogue J, Sheridan P, Dinccag N, Hanefeld M, Hoogwerf B, Laakso M, Mohan V, Shaw J, Zinman B, Holman RR. Effect of rosiglitazone on the frequency of diabetes in patients with impaired glucose tolerance or impaired fasting glucose: a randomised controlled trial. Lancet 2006; 368:1096–105.

ELSEVIER

International Congress Series 1303 (2007) 146–154

www.ics-elsevier.com

The blockade of the endocannabinoid CB1 receptors and its influence on cardiometabolic risk: Lesson from Rimonabant In Obesity (RIO) trials

Roberto Vettor *, Marco Rossato, Francesco Fallo, Claudio Pagano

Endocrine-metabolic laboratory, Internal Medicine 3, Department of Medical and Surgical Sciences, University of Padova, via Ospedale 105, 35128 Padova, Italy

Abstract. The impact of visceral obesity epidemic on the incidence of diabetes mellitus and cardiovascular disease is a major concern in the public health management. Even if lifestyle modifications still remain the cornerstone of obesity treatment, the pharmacological approach could help not only to reduce body weight and visceral fat but also their metabolic and cardiovascular complications. It has been shown that endogenous cannabinoid system is overactivated in obese mice and both in subcutaneous and visceral adipose tissue of obese patients. The CB1 antagonist rimonabant is able to antagonize most of the behavioural and metabolic effect of endocannabinoid overactivation. Four double-blind trials compared rimonabant 5 mg or 20 mg daily with placebo in more than 6600 individuals. RIO-Europe, RIO-Lipids, RIO-North America, and RIO-Diabetes have published 1 year results. RIO-North America also included a second year of follow-up. These trials showed that in patients with obesity, including those with cardiovascular risk factors, continued therapy with rimonabant as compared with placebo is associated with a significant reduction in body weight and waist circumference. Such therapy is also associated with other favorable changes in the cardiometabolic risk profile, including an improvement in the lipid profile and in glycaemic control in type 2 diabetics. © 2007 Published by Elsevier B.V.

Keywords: Obesity; Type 2 diabetes; Endocannabinoids; Rimonabant; Clinical trials

Cardiovascular disease still remains the most important cause of morbidity and mortality in the developed countries. Obesity is a major concern with epidemic proportions and it has been reported that in the upcoming years a terrible impact of the obesity epidemic on the incidence

* Corresponding author.
E-mail address: roberto.vettor@unipd.it (R. Vettor).

0531-5131/ © 2007 Published by Elsevier B.V.
doi:10.1016/j.ics.2007.03.025

of diabetes mellitus and cardiovascular disease will be expected. Expansion of the adipose organ, and in particular of visceral depots, increases the risk of obesity complications (i.e. insulin resistance, type 2 diabetes, atherosclerosis, steatohepatitis, cardio- and cerebrovascular diseases). Obesity is the major pathophysiological clustering factor of the clinically useful, but not yet pathophysiologically defined, metabolic syndrome which is associated with an increased risk of mortality. Primary prevention of each metabolic syndrome condition and in particular of visceral obesity should be stressed. At present there is strong scientific evidence that energy fuel overflow with subsequent enlargement of adipose tissue represents the key pathophysiological starting point. Adipose tissue secretes a variety of adipokines, that contribute to insulin resistance, endothelial dysfunction, and atherogenesis [1]. This fact may explain the coexistence of adipose tissue enlargement with glucose intolerance, dyslipidaemia, low grade chronic inflammation and hypertension. The last National Cholesterol Education Program (Adult Treatment Panel III) stipulative definition of the metabolic syndrome [2], help us to identify individuals with a strikingly elevated risk of developing diabetes and atherosclerosis with their potential complications like myocardial infarction and stroke. Therefore any effort we can put forward in order to modify the cardiometabolic risk factors, and in particular abdominal obesity, will have definite favourable effect on lipid profile, blood pressure, blood glucose and C-reactive protein and a decrease in mortality [3]. However, results with the behavioural therapy and currently available drugs in achieving significant and persistent weight loss are quite limited. Bariatric surgery, such as gastric banding or gastric bypass, despite its effectiveness in morbid obese people, is neither a feasible nor a desirable population-based treatment for obesity.

1.1. The endocannabinoid system

The most important psychoactive natural compound present in the plant *cannabis sativa* is the Δ^9-tetrahydrocannabinol which was used extensively in the eastern traditional medicine to improve appetite in chronic diseases. The endogenous cannabinoid system has been demonstrated to be an important regulator of energy homeostasis acting through central pathways whose endogenous ligands (2-arachidonoylglycerol and anandamide) activate the type 1 cannabinoid receptor (CB1). Under normal conditions, the endocannabinoid system is not tonically active; rather endocannabinoids are produced on demand, act locally, and are rapidly inactivated via cellular uptake and enzymatic hydrolysis [4]. The cannabinoids exert their physiological actions not only through the interaction with the CB_1, but also with the specific receptor CB_2 [5]. The CB_1 receptors are primarily distributed in the brain and adipose tissue, but are also found in the myocardium, vascular endothelium, and sympathetic nerve terminals. The CB_2 receptors are primarily located in the immune cells. Both receptors function as transmembrane G-coupled receptors. The existence of a CB_3 receptors has been postulated, but has not yet been cloned.

There is increasing evidence showing that the endocannabinoid system plays a central role in regulating metabolism and body composition by enhancing the central orexigenic drive and increasing peripheral lipogenesis [6,7]. Control of food intake and body composition is the result of a series of complex interactions between the adipocytes, the mesolimbic system, the hypothalamus, and the gastrointestinal tract. There is now evidence that both cannabinoid receptors and their endogenous ligands are present in the CNS and play an important role in the regulation of food intake. Levels of endocannabinoids in the hypothalamus are decreased after administration of leptin [8]. The CB_1 agonists are potent, dose-dependent inducers of hyperphagia in rodents [9], and antagonism of CB_1 receptors prevents hyperphagia in a starvation model [8]. CB1 knockout mice display decreased body fat and are resistant to diet-induced obesity showing also a lower plasma insulin levels and a higher sensitivity to leptin [10]. Evidence is accumulating to indicate that the endogenous cannabinoid system is present also in peripheral tissues. Enzymatic pathways for the synthesis of endogenous cannabinoids and CB1 receptors are expressed in peripheral tissues involved in energy metabolism (liver, adipose tissue, skeletal muscle). Activation of CB1 receptors in the liver was shown to increase de novo synthesis of fatty acids by activating the transcription factor sterol regulatory element-binding protein 1c (SREBP-1c) in mice [11]. CB1 is upregulated in adipose tissue of genetically obese Zucker rats and treatment with the CB1 antagonist SR141716 increases the expression of adiponectin both in vivo in mice and in vitro in 3T3-F442A cells. However most of the peripheral effects of cannabinoids were reported in rodents and in cell lines while the role of the endocannabinoid system in humans has been by far less investigated. Endogenous cannabinoids are increased both in subcutaneous and visceral adipose tissue of obese patients and in diet-induced obese mice [12–14]. However no direct evidence has been reported so far on the direct effects of endocannabinoids on glucose and lipid metabolism and on adiponectin release in human fat cells.

1.2. Rimonabant

Rimonabant was the first CB1-receptor blocker described in 1994 by Rinaldi-Carmona et al. [15]. It displays a 1000-fold greater affinity for the CB1 than for the CB2 receptor and blocks calcium and potassium channels [16]. The drug is metabolised in the liver and excreted in bile. Because of a larger peripheral volume of distribution, obese individuals have a drug half-life that is twice as long (16 days) as non-obese people. Rimonabant produces a dose-dependent reduction in food intake in various rodent models and this effect seem to be both centrally and peripherally mediated. Potential peripheral mechanisms include enhanced thermogenesis via increased oxygen consumption in skeletal muscle, diminished hepatic and adipocyte lipogenesis, augmentation of adiponectin concentrations, promotion of vagally mediated cholecystokin-induced satiety, inhibition of preadipocyte proliferation, and increased adipocyte maturation without lipid accumulation [12].

1.3. Rimonabant for treatment of obesity and cardiometabolic risk factors: animal data

The impact of CB_1 antagonist rimonabant on food intake and body weight was firstly investigated in animal models by Di Marzo et al. [8] who showed that this drug was associated with a reduction in food intake and a significant loss of body weight in wild-type mice, but not in CB_1 receptor-deficient mice. The decrease in visceral adipose tissue accounted for most of the rimonabant-induced weight loss, with the muscle mass remaining unchanged or even increased [13]. It has also been reported [17] that in diet-induced obese mice, treatment with the CB_1 antagonist was associated with a remarkable and persistent weight reduction with a clear improvement in insulin sensitivity, despite a reduction in food intake that was only transient. Rimonabant was also shown to increase both adiponectin gene expression in the adipocytes and adiponectin plasma levels [14]. These findings strongly suggest the existence of a CB_1-mediated mechanism of the anti-obesity action of rimonabant at the adipose tissue level.

2. Rimonabant In Obesity (RIO) trials

Four double-blind trials, included in the Rimonabant In Obesity (RIO) Program, compared rimonabant 5 mg or 20 mg daily with placebo in more than 6600 individuals. RIO-Europe, RIO-Lipids, RIO-North America, and RIO-Diabetes have published 1 year results. RIO-North America also included a second year of follow-up in which rimonabant-treated patients were re-randomized to continue active drug treatment or switched to placebo [18] The RIO Program enrolled patients with BMI of 30 kg/m^2 or greater or BMI higher than 27 kg/m^2 with dyslipidaemia (predominantly high triglyceride or low HDL cholesterol concentrations), type 2 diabetes, or hypertension. The 5 mg dose of rimonabant had little efficacy and therefore we will focus on the results with 20 mg.

2.1. The RIO-Lipids trial

The RIO-Lipids trial enrolled 1036 patients [19] for one year. Rimonabant administration was associated with significantly greater weight loss compared to placebo at the end of one-year treatment. A substantial ≥10% weight loss was sustained by 32.6% of subjects in the high-dose rimonabant group, compared with 10.6% in the low-dose group and 7.2% in the placebo group. Another important aim of this study was to analyze the weight loss-dependent or -independent drug-induced changes in the lipid profile (Fig. 1).

During treatment, triglycerides remained stable in the placebo group, but fell 15.8±8.0% in the group receiving 20 mg of rimonabant. HDL cholesterol increased in a dose-dependent fashion, achieving an increase of 23.4±1.8% in the group receiving 20 mg of rimonabant. Although there was no change in levels of LDL cholesterol, the distribution of LDL particles

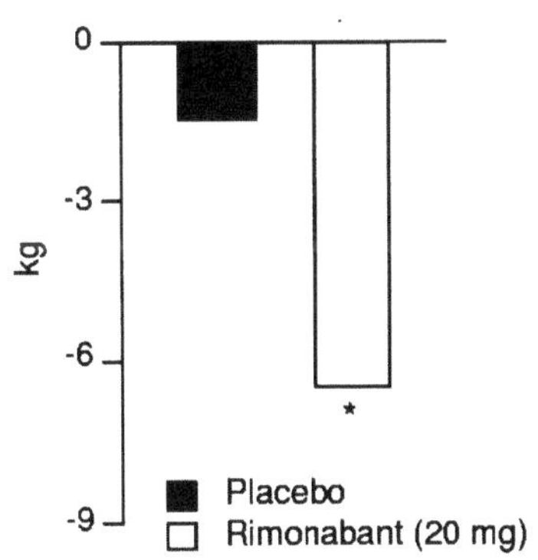

Fig. 1. Mean body weight reduction after 1 year treatment with placebo or rimonabant 20 mg in the 4 RIO trials (RIO-Lipids, RIO-North America, RIO-Europe and RIO-Diabetes).

shifted toward larger size in the group receiving 20 mg of rimonabant, as compared with placebo, with a difference of 4.6% lower proportion of small dense LDL particles.

The C-reactive protein levels were lower in the high-dose rimonabant group (27% reduction vs. 11% for placebo), and the low-density lipoprotein (LDL) levels were not significantly affected by treatment. Rimonabant 20 mg also increased adiponectin levels by 57.7%, a change that was partly independent of weight loss. Levels of fasting plasma insulin, the one-hour and two-hour plasma glucose and insulin levels, and the insulin and glucose AUCs during the 75-grams oral glucose-tolerance test decreased significantly in the group receiving 20 mg of rimonabant.

2.2. *The RIO-Europe trial*

1507 subjects were enrolled in the RIO-Europe trial [20] and assigned randomly to receive rimonabant 20 mg/day, rimonabant 5 mg/day, or placebo. Subjects were also given instructions for moderate physical exercise and a mild hypocaloric diet. Among patients completing one full year of treatment (61%) placebo-subtracted analysis showed that rimonabant 20 mg was associated with significant weight loss and reduction in waist circumference. Triglyceride levels decreased and HDL levels increased in both rimonabant groups. Rimonabant treatment was associated with significant improvements in lipid and glycaemic variables. Importantly, the improvements in HDL cholesterol and triglycerides observed in this study could not be fully explained by the observed weight loss alone. In fact the weight-loss-adjusted difference in HDL cholesterol (expressed as the percentage change from baseline) between the placebo and rimonabant 20 mg groups was 3.6%, compared with an unadjusted difference of 8.9%; this value would translate to about 60% of the increase in HDL cholesterol being accounted for by the observed weight loss in the ITT population. Similarly, the weight-loss-adjusted difference in the percentage change in triglyceride concentrations between placebo and rimonabant 20 mg was −8.3% compared with the unadjusted difference of −15.1% in the ITT population, corresponding to about 45% of the reduction being accounted for by the observed weight loss. A possible explanation for the potential weight-independent effect of rimonabant on HDL cholesterol and triglycerides might be related to the observation that rimonabant enhances the mRNA expression of adiponectin, an adipokine secreted by fat cells and reported to have a role in the regulation of hyperglycaemia, hyperinsulinaemia, and fatty acid oxidation [1].

2.3. *The RIO-North America trial*

Obese patients in North America (NA) were enrolled into the RIO-North America (NA) trial [21]. In addition to evaluating the efficacy of rimonabant for primary weight loss, this 3045-subject trial had evaluated whether weight loss achieved with rimonabant could be maintained after withdrawal of the drug. In this study after the completion of one year of treatment, subjects in the two rimonabant groups underwent a second randomization, either to continue receiving their previously assigned dose of rimonabant or to be switched to placebo. The first-year outcomes were similar to those of the other RIO trials: weight loss was significantly greater in the rimonabant treatment groups (−6.3 kg for 20 mg/day vs −1.6 kg for placebo). After two years, subjects re-randomized to placebo after the end of one year have regained much of their weight (overall loss of 3.2 kg vs. 2.3 kg for patients on placebo for two years), whereas those who were treated with rimonabant 20 mg/day for the full two years lost an average of 7.4 kg. An increase in HDL of 24.5% was seen in the rimonabant 20 mg/day group, compared with 13.8% in the placebo group.

2.4. The RIO-Diabetes trial

The most recent study reported from the RIO phase 3 program was the RIO-Diabetes trial [22]. This multicentre randomized controlled trial was designed to assess the efficacy and safety of rimonabant in combination with a mild hypocaloric diet and advice for increased physical activity in overweight or obese patients with type 2 diabetes who were already on metformin or sulphonylurea monotherapy for at least 6 months (stable dose for at least 3 months).

This study enrolled 1047 patients with type 2 diabetes mellitus and a BMI of 27 to 40 kg/m^2, haemoglobin A1c (HbA1c) level of 6.5–10.0%, and fasting glucose concentration of 5.55–15.04 mmol/L. Again, subjects were randomized to receive rimonabant 20 mg/day, rimonabant 5 mg/day, or placebo for one year.

An average weight loss of 5.3 kg, compared with 1.4 kg in the placebo group from baseline at the last observation carried forward (LOCF) at the end of one year therapy with rimonabant 20 mg was observed. Average levels of HbA1c were decreased by 0.6% in the rimonabant 20 mg group from a baseline level of 7.3%, but were increased in the placebo group by 0.1% ($p<0.001$). Importantly, 43% of all subjects treated with rimonabant achieved an optimal HbA1c level of <6.5%, compared with only 21% of those receiving placebo. The observed effects of 20 mg/day rimonabant on HbA1c were about twice that attributable to concurrent weight loss alone.

A significant amelioration of secondary endpoints including waist circumference, blood pressure and changes in HDL cholesterol, triglyceride, fasting glucose, fasting insulin, high-sensitivity C-reactive protein (hsCRP), and leptin concentrations was reported. It is important to note that the residual effect on HDL cholesterol concentration of 20 mg/day rimonabant was 57% of the observed effect after adjustment for weight loss. The residual effect on triglyceride concentration after adjustment for weight loss was 36% of the observed effect, which was not significant. Insulin resistance index calculated by use of the homoeostasis model assessment (HOMA-IR) was clearly decreased. Effects of the rimonabant 5 mg/day were less significant. Besides the improvement of glycaemic control in the reduction of microvascular and macrovascular complications, considerable emphasis has been placed on aggressive management of multiple cardiovascular and metabolic risk factors in type 2 diabetes patients. In the RIO-Diabetes rimonabant not only improved the atherogenic dyslipidaemia, but also diminished systolic blood pressure in diabetic patients, and reduced the persisting prevalence of the metabolic syndrome assessed in accordance with NCEP-ATP III criteria, as in the RIO-Lipid study. Compared with placebo, 20 mg/day rimonabant also reduced hsCRP, the inflammatory biomarker which is considered a forecaster of cardiovascular disease.

Health-related quality of life was specifically assessed with IWQoL-Lite. A greater improvement at 1 year in the physical function and self-esteem domains and in the total IWQoL-Lite score was noted in the 20 mg/day rimonabant group than in the placebo group.

In summary, the RIO trials showed that in patients with obesity, including those with cardiovascular risk factors, continued therapy with rimonabant as compared with placebo is associated with a significant reduction in body weight and waist circumference. Such therapy is also associated with other favorable changes in the cardiometabolic risk profile, including an improvement in glycaemic control in type 2 diabetics and the lipid profile. In the four trials an important final finding was that at the end of treatment, the proportion of patients satisfying the National Cholesterol Education Program-Adult Treatment Panel III criteria for metabolic syndrome was significantly lower in the high-dose rimonabant-treated group compared with placebo (Fig. 2).

2.5. Adverse effects in clinical trials of rimonabant

Initial experience with rimonabant shows that it is generally well tolerated. In the RIO phase 3 program, the one-year dropout rates were high (36% to 49%), but were typical of obesity trials and did not differ from placebo. A slightly greater proportion of patients in the rimonabant treatment groups experienced adverse events than did those in the placebo group. The most common adverse events, occurring in 5% or more rimonabant-treated patients, were nausea, diarrhoea, vomiting, dizziness, hypoglycaemia, fatigue. The most common adverse events that led to premature study discontinuation in the 20 mg/day rimonabant group were

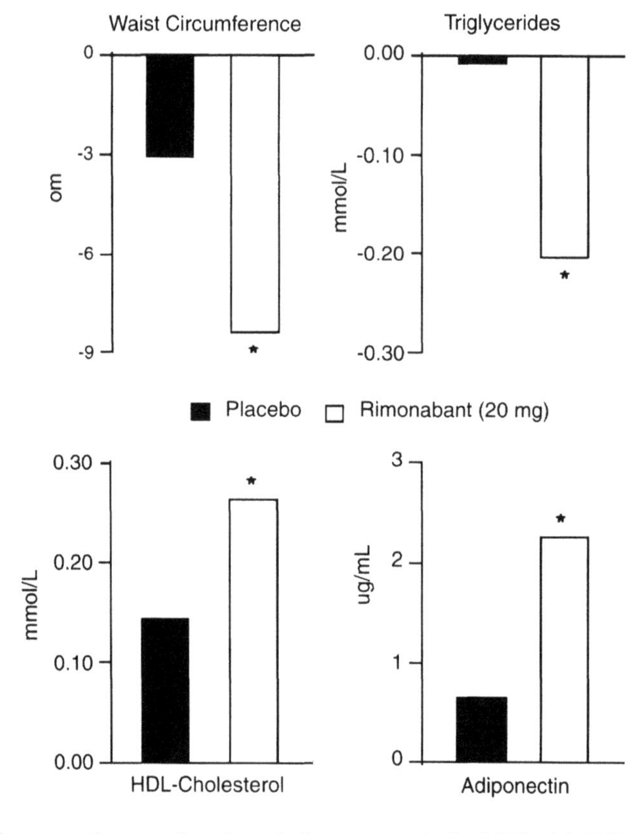

Fig. 2. Changes in some anthropometric and metabolic parameters in the 3 RIO trials (RIO-Lipids, RIO-North America, RIO-Europe).

anxiety and depressed mood disorders, nausea, and dizziness. These were generally mild or moderate, transient and self-limited, and were seen early in the treatment period. However, no serious adverse events linked to psychiatric disorders were recorded in either rimonabant group. Use of the Hospital Anxiety and Depression scale in RIO-Europe showed no difference between the treatment groups in the average subscale scores for either major depression or anxiety. During one year of treatment, six subjects (1.0%) in the rimonabant 20 mg/day group and one subject (0.3%) in the placebo group discontinued their study drug because of depression. For depressed mood disorders, the rates were 3.7% and 3.0% for rimonabant 20 mg/day and placebo respectively. Similarly, in RIO-Lipids, the Hospital Anxiety and Depression scale scores were similar for anxiety and depression between the two treatment groups and placebo. Therefore, it seems that the percentage of patients experiencing neuropsychiatric side effects is small. Monitoring for on-treatment anxiety and depression in the future will nonetheless be necessary to ensure safe use of this new therapy.

2.6. Clinical applications and the ideal patient profile

The failure in the obesity drug treatment in the long term weight loss maintenance is probably related to the hypersimplification of the obesity phenotype and the consequent therapeutic choice. Obese subjects may have either a visceral or a peripheral fat distribution, they may be actually overeaters or simply sedentary, diabetic or not, hypertensive or not. The complexity of clinical signs and symptoms could be useful in defining the precise target and to utilize a selective drug. Rimonabant may be considered a good choice in visceral obese patients with an atherogenic lipid profile (low HDL cholesterol and high triglyceride concentrations) associated with metabolic syndrome. The drug should be used with caution, or should be avoided, in patients with pre-existing psychiatric illness, particularly depression or anxiety, and in those with liver impairment. Treatment should be discontinued if clinically significant weight loss (i.e. at least 5–10% of initial body weight or improvement in major obesity-related comorbidity) does not occur within the first 3 months. Furthermore, the optimum long-term duration of treatment is supported by efficacy and safety data of only 2 years clinical trials and therefore we are not allowed to consider equally safe a longer period of treatment until new long-term data will be available from clinical trials or post marketing drug survey.

Finally the lack of cardiovascular morbidity and mortality endpoints in obesity drug trials represents a major gap in knowledge. Surrogate endpoints such as weight loss might not necessarily improve endpoints judged to be more clinically relevant. In the RIO trials rimonabant also significantly reduced the placebo-subtracted incidence of metabolic syndrome in all four trials and the placebo-subtracted HbA1c by 0.7% in RIO-Diabetes. Concentrations of LDL cholesterol did not improve, but an amelioration in the atherogenic lipid profile was always present. Compared with placebo, blood pressure was either unchanged or slightly reduced.

Even if no data on cardiovascular morbidity or mortality have been reported so far, several rimonabant studies examining clinical endpoints and surrogate measurements of atherosclerotic burden (eg, intravascular ultrasound) are underway. The largest is the Comprehensive Rimonabant Evaluation Study of Cardiovascular Endpoints and Outcomes (CRESCENDO) trial, which is investigating the effect of rimonabant on myocardial infarction, stroke and cardiovascular death in 17,000 obese participants (NCT 00263042 *www.ClinicalTrials.gov*).

References

[1] R. Vettor, G. Milan, M. Rossato, Federspil review article: adipocytokines and insulin resistance, Aliment. Pharmacol. Ther. 22 (Suppl 2) (2005) 3–10.

[2] Executive Summary of the Third Report of the National Cholesterol Education Program (NCEP) Expert panel on detection, evaluation, and treatment of high blood cholesterol in adults (Adult Treatment Panel III), JAMA 285 (2001) 2486–2497.

[3] T.A. Wadden, D.A. Anderson, G.D. Foster, Two-year changes in lipids and lipoproteins associated with the maintenance of a 5% to 10% reduction in initial weight some findings and some questions, Obes. Res. 7 (1999) 170–178.

[4] A. Giuffrida, M. Beltramo, D. Piomelli, Mechanisms of endocannabinoid inactivation biochemistry and pharmacology, J. Pharmacol. Exp. Ther. 298 (2001) 7–14.

[5] S. Munro, K.L. Thomas, M. Abu-Shaar, Molecular characterization of a peripheral receptor for cannabinoids, Nature 365 (1993) 61–65.

[6] D. Cota, et al., The endogenous cannabinoid system affects energy balance via central orexigenic drive and peripheral lipogenesis, J. Clin. Invest. 112 (3) (2003) 423–431.

[7] D. Cota, et al., The endogenous cannabinoid system affects energy balance via central orexigenic drive and peripheral lipogenesis, J. Clin. Invest. 112 (2003) 423–431.

[8] V. Di Marzo, et al., Leptin-regulated endocannabinoids are involved in maintaining food intake, Nature 410 (2001) 822–825.

[9] T.C. Kirkham, et al., Endocannabinoid levels in rat limbic forebrain and hypothalamus in relation to fasting, feeding and satiation stimulation of eating by 2-arachidonoyl glycerol, Br. J. Pharmacol. 136 (2002) 550–557.

[10] C. Ravinet, et al., CB1 cannabinoid receptor knockout in mice leads to leanness, resistance to diet-induced obesity and enhanced leptin sensitivity, Int. J. Obes. Relat. Metab. Disord. 28 (2004) 640–648.

[11] D. Osei-Hyiaman, et al., Endocannabinoid activation at hepatic CB1 receptors stimulates fatty acid synthesis and contributes to diet-induced obesity, J. Clin. Invest. 115 (5) (2005) 1298–1305.

[12] S. Engeli, J. Jordan, The endocannabinoid system: body weight and metabolic regulation, Clin. Cornerstone 8 (Suppl 4) (2006) S24–S35.

[13] O. Jbilo, et al., The CB1 receptor antagonist rimonabant reverses the diet-induced obesity phenotype through the regulation of lipolysis and energy balance, FASEB J. 19 (2005) 1567–1569.

[14] M. Bensaid, et al., The cannabinoid CB1 receptor antagonist SR141716 increases Acrp30 mRNA expression in adipose tissue of obese fa/fa rats and in cultured adipocyte cells, Mol. Pharmacol. 63 (2003) 908–914.

[15] M. Rinaldi-Carmona, et al., SR141716A, a potent and selective antagonist of the brain cannabinoid receptor, FEBS Lett. 350 (1994) 240–244.

[16] R. White, C.R. Hiley, The actions of the cannabinoid receptor antagonist, SR 141716A, in the rat isolated mesenteric artery, Br. J. Pharmacol. 125 (1998) 689–696.

[17] C. Ravinet-Trillou, et al., Anti-obesity effect of SR141716, a CB1 receptor antagonist, in diet-induced obese mice, Am. J. Physiol., Regul. Integr. Comp. Physiol. 284 (2003) R345–R353.

[18] E.V. Gelfand, C.P. Cannon, Rimonabant: a cannabinoid receptor type 1 blocker for management of multiple cardiometabolic risk factors, J. Am. Coll. Cardiol. 47 (10) (2006) 1919–1926.

[19] J.P. Despres, A. Golay, L. Sjostrom, Effects of rimonabant on metabolic risk factors in overweight patients with dyslipidemia, N. Engl. J. Med. 353 (2005) 2121–2134.

[20] L.F. VanGaal, et al., Effects of the cannabinoid-1 receptor blocker rimonabant on weight reduction and cardiovascular risk factors in overweight patients 1-year experience from the RIO-Europe study, Lancet 365 (2005) 1389–1397.

[21] F.X. Pi-Sunyer, et al., Effect of rimonabant, a cannabinoid-1 receptor blocker, on weight and cardiometabolic risk factors in overweight or obese patients: RIO-North America: a randomized controlled trial, JAMA 295 (2006) 761–775.

[22] A.J. Scheen, et al., Efficacy and tolerability of rimonabant in overweight or obese patients with type 2 diabetes: a randomised controlled study, Lancet 368 (9548) (2006) 1660–1672.

ELSEVIER

International Congress Series 1303 (2007) 155–159

www.ics-elsevier.com

Efficacy and safety of pioglitazone: The proactive study

Paolo Brunetti *

Department of Internal Medicine, University of Perugia, Via Enrico dal Pozzo, 06126 Perugia, Italy

Abstract. In this paper a new analysis of the PROactive study is presented. If procedure-related endpoints (coronary and leg revascularisation) are excluded, the efficacy of pioglitazone in the prevention of all-cause mortality, non-fatal myocardial infarction and stroke, in high risk type 2 diabetic patients, is clearly shown by the study. As far as the safety issues are concerned, the reported increase in heart failure is most likely due to the greater incidence of edema in pioglitazone-treated patients. © 2007 Published by Elsevier B.V.

Keywords: PROactive study; Type 2 diabetes; Pioglitazone; Myocardial infarction; Heart failure

1. Introduction

The UKPDS has demonstrated that glucose control has a dramatic impact on the prevention of microangiopathy but only a moderate and not significant effect on cardiovascular complications [1].

On the other hand, pioglitazone has been accredited with a series of extrahypoglycemic, potentially anti-atherosclerotic and cardioprotective effects [2].

The PROactive study (PROspective pioglitAzone Clinical Trial In macroVascular Events) was therefore designed to investigate whether pioglitazone, when added on top of preexisting therapy, was able to reduce total mortality and macrovascular morbidity in a high risk population of type 2 diabetic patients [3].

* Tel.: +39 075 5783747; fax: +39 075 5730855.
E-mail address: pabrunet@unipg.it.

0531-5131/ © 2007 Published by Elsevier B.V.
doi:10.1016/j.ics.2007.03.018

2. Study design

The study was planned to recruit 5000 patients, with a minimum of 2.5 years exposure to treatment and a minimum of 760 patients with one or more cardiovascular events, and had a 91% power to detect a 20% reduction in the hazard rate.

The main inclusion criteria were an HbA1c concentration above the upper limit of normal (6.5% according to IDF) and a well-established history of macrovascular disease, defined as one or more atherosclerotic complications.

The population included in the trial was therefore at very high risk of cardiovascular events: almost 50% of the 5238 patients enrolled in the study had a prior history of myocardial infarction and almost 20% a prior history of stroke and, again, almost 50% of the patients had 2 or more entry criteria as it is also shown by the frequent overlap in the same subjects of different macrovascular diseases.

The primary endpoint of the study was a composite one, including both disease-related endpoints, like all-cause mortality, non-fatal myocardial infarction, stroke, leg amputations and acute coronary syndrome, and procedure-related endpoints, like coronary and leg revascularisation.

The procedure-related endpoints were included to increase the probability of an adequate number of events in the composite primary endpoint, but the first three components of the composite, with the exception of silent myocardial infarction, were also selected to constitute the predefined principal secondary endpoint.

In effect, mortality, myocardial infarction and stroke are hard endpoints and, moreover, independent from the technology availability and the decision making of the different recruiting centres.

3. Results: pioglitazone efficacy

The results of the study have been the object of an intense debate. In fact, the primary endpoint was not reached: patients treated with pioglitazone had only a 10% risk reduction, which, however, did not reach statistical significance.

One possible reason for such result is the shorter duration of the trial due to the faster recruitment than originally expected. It is possible that a delayed closure of the trial would have allowed to reach the statistical significance. But the main reason is to be found in the heterogeneous composition of the primary endpoint itself. In fact, when we consider the principal secondary endpoint, which includes only disease-related endpoints, the relative risk reduction of death, myocardial infarction and stroke was 16% and the result is highly significant.

In Table 1 the number of first events contributing to the primary composite and main secondary endpoints is shown. Both in the primary and secondary endpoints, patients treated with pioglitazone had a clear reduction of death, myocardial infarction and stroke. Also the number of amputations and of acute coronary syndrome are reduced.

This is not true, on the contrary, for the procedure-related endpoints, coronary and leg revascularisation. Therefore, when these events are excluded, as in the predefined principal secondary endpoint, the difference between the two groups becomes still more evident.

Table 1
Numbers of first events contributing to the primary composite and principal secondary endpoints (from Dormandy et al. [3])

	Primary composite endpoint		Principal secondary endpoint	
	Piog, n=2605	Pbo, n=2633	Piog, n=2605	Pbo, n=2633
Any endpoint	514	572	301	358
Death	110	122	129	142
Non-fatal MI (excluding silent MI)	85	95	90	116
Silent MI	20	23	–	–
Stroke	76	96	82	100
Major leg amputations	9	15	–	–
Acute coronary syndrome	42	63	–	–
Coronary revascularisation	101	101	–	–
Leg revascularisation	71	57	–	–

MI: myocardial infarction.

A multivariate analysis of the association of entry characteristics to the main secondary endpoint has shown that most factors considered at baseline, age, smoke, previous myocardial infarction or stroke, HbA1c, but also insulin therapy, metformin and sulphonylurea treatment, HDL-C and triglycerides, are associated with a highly significant risk. On the contrary, allocation to pioglitazone is associated with a HR of 0.84 even after adjustment for the other factors in this table.

So, in spite of the fact that the primary endpoint was not reached, we can agree with the official statement of ADA according to which "there appeared to be a clear benefit of adding pioglitazone to type 2 diabetic patients already using most of the conventional classes of glucose-lowering agents" [4].

These conclusions were further supported by the analysis of subgroups of patients. In particular, in patients with previous myocardial infarction, the recurrence of fatal and non-fatal myocardial infarction, excluding silent myocardial infarction, was prevented in 28% of cases [5].

Similar results have been presented in Copenhagen at the EASD meeting. Pioglitazone group has shown a risk reduction of 23% for myocardial infarction and a risk reduction of 17% for major cardiovascular events (MACE2) defined as all-cause mortality, non-fatal myocardial infarction (excluding silent myocardial infarction), non-fatal stroke or acute coronary syndrome [6].

Moreover, in a prespecified subgroup analysis, pioglitazone-treated patients with previous stroke had a highly significant benefit in terms of a new stroke prevention with a risk reduction of 47%. In the same subjects there was also a clear reduction in a composite endpoint of major cardiovascular events and in all causes of death [7].

Concomitant medications did not change during the trial with the only exception of metformin and insulin which rose more – particularly insulin – in the placebo group. At the end of the study, insulin therapy was adopted permanently in the pioglitazone group by a number of patients which was less than half the number of patients who needed insulin in the placebo group [3]. There is only one possible explanation of these data and it is that thiazolidinediones have a sparing effect on β-cells as, on the other hand, has been demonstrated in several clinical and animal studies [8,9].

We can find a further proof of this concept in the stable reduction of HbA1c without any rebound during the trial [3], as it was observed instead during the UKPDS, since the first year, due to the progressive decline of beta-cell function [1].

If the progression of type 2 diabetes is due to the progressive loss of beta-cell mass [10], pioglitazone seems to stop or to delay this process through an antiapoptotic effect.

Besides improving blood glucose control, pioglitazone has a positive effect on HDL-C, blood pressure and triglycerides. None of these effects, however, can explain per se the cardiovascular protection induced by pioglitazone during the trial.

Even if inflammatory markers were not measured during the study, the antiinflammatory effects of TZD have been thoroughly demonstrated in a wide series of other clinical and experimental investigations [2].

4. Results: pioglitazone safety

Since the first presentation of the study in Athens, the safety issues have been the subject of a wide debate. In particular, the higher reported rate of heart failure and of hospitalisation due to heart failure has been a cause of big concern.

But it should be stressed that despite the increase in reported heart failure in the pioglitazone group, the number of deaths from heart failure was similar in each group and, therefore, the most likely explanation is that heart failure has been overdiagnosed because of the increased incidence of edema in pioglitazone-treated patients. In fact, the mortality of diabetic patients with heart failure is so high, in comparison with non-diabetics [11], that there is no other way to explain the discrepancy between reported heart failure and number of deaths.

Moreover, the clinical diagnosis of heart failure is not so easy to be established, being validated in a small percentage of patients as it is shown by several studies [12,13]. Such conclusions can be easily applied to the PROactive study because the episodes of heart failure were diagnosed by the investigators but were not adjudicated centrally by the Endpoint Adjudication Committee.

The relationship between diabetes, heart failure and anti-hyperglycemic therapy can also be considered from a different point of view. Diabetic patients are particularly prone to heart failure but it is also true that heart failure is not only the effect but also a cause of diabetes. Heart failure is indeed an independent risk factor for the development of insulin resistance and diabetes and the risk increases with the severity of heart failure.

This explains why patients admitted to the hospital because of heart failure and treated, after discharge, with a thiazolidinedione (rosiglitazone or pioglitazone), having refused insulin therapy, presented a significant reduction of mortality [14]. The same is true for metformin and still better results have been obtained with a relative risk reduction of 48%, with the combination of metformin and a thiazolidinedione [15].

We could agree, therefore, with the joint statement of AHA and ADA, according to which thiazolidinediones should not be used in NYHA III–IV class heart failure, but might be used instead, cautiously, with initiation of treatment at the lowest dose and gradual dose escalation, in NYHA I–II class patients. In Europe, only NYHA class I patients are admitted to glitazone therapy.

No other relevant adverse events were observed besides a moderate increase in peripheral edema and an average weight gain of 3.6 kg.

No increase in malignancy and liver toxicity were observed. There was instead a net decrease of serum transaminase activity certainly due to the reduction of lipid storage in the liver.

5. Conclusions

In conclusion, the PROactive study has demonstrated for the first time that a glucose-lowering medication can prevent macrovascular events in high risk patients with type 2 diabetes. In particular, pioglitazone reduces the composite of all-cause mortality, non-fatal myocardial infarction and stroke. Adding pioglitazone to the medications of 1000 patients would avoid 21 first myocardial infarctions, strokes or deaths over 3 years. In other words, 48 patients would need to be treated for 3 years to avoid one first major cardiovascular event.

Finally pioglitazone decreases the need for conversion to insulin therapy and its use in type 2 diabetic patients should be considered substantially safe.

References

[1] UK Prospective Diabetes Study (UKPDS) Group, Intensive blood-glucose control with sulphonylureas or insulin compared with conventional treatment and risk of complications inpatients with type 2 diabetes (UKPDS 33), Lancet 352 (1998) 837–853.

[2] B. Staels, PPARγ and atherosclerosis, Curr. Med. Res. Opin. 21 (Suppl. 1) (2005) S13–S20.

[3] J.A. Dormandy, et al., Secondary prevention of macrovascular events in patients with type 2 diabetes in the PROactive study (Prospective pioglitAzone Clinical Trial In Macrovascular Events): a randomized controlled trial, Lancet 366 (2005) 1279–1289.

[4] R. Rizza, R. Henry, R. Kahn, Commentary on the results and clinical implications of the PROactive study, Diabetes Care 28 (2005) 2965–2967.

[5] E. Erdmann, Pioglitazone treatment in patients with type 2 diabetes and a history of MI: subgroup analyses from PROactive stratified by gender, age, and duration of diabetes, Presented at the Congress of the European Association for the Study of Diabetes, Copenhagen, September 14–17 2006.

[6] R. Wilcox, on behalf of the PROactive investigators, An analysis from PROactive on the effect of pioglitazone on major adverse cardiovascular events (MACE) and myocardial infarction, Presented at the Congress of the European Association for the Study of Diabetes, Copenhagen, September 14–17 2006.

[7] J.A. Dormandy, M.G. Bousser, R. Wilcox, Pioglitazone in patients with or without a history of stroke: results from PROactive, Presented at the Congress of the European Association for the Study of Diabetes, Copenhagen, 14–17 September 2006.

[8] T.A. Buchanan, et al., Preservation of pancreatic [beta]-cell function and prevention of type 2 diabetes by pharmacological treatment of insulin resistance in high-risk hispanic women, Diabetes 51 (2002) 2796–2803.

[9] D.T. Finegood, et al., [beta]-Cell mass dynamics in Zucker diabetic fatty rats: rosiglitazone prevents the rise in net cell death, Diabetes 50 (2001) 1021–1029.

[10] A.E. Butler, et al., [beta]-Cell deficit and increased [beta]-cell apoptosis in humans with type 2 diabetes, Diabetes 52 (2003) 102–110.

[11] G.A. Nichols, et al., Congestive heart failure in type 2 diabetes: prevalence, incidence, and risk factors, Diabetes Care 24 (2001) 1614–1619.

[12] J. Remes, et al., Validity of clinical diagnosis of heart failure in primary health care, Eur. Heart J. 12 (1991) 315–321.

[13] M.R. Cowie, et al., Aetiology of heart failure: a population based study, Eur. Heart J. 20 (1999) 421–428.

[14] F.A. Masoudi, et al., Thiazolidinediones, metformin, and outcomes in older patients with diabetes and heart failure. An observational study, Circulation 111 (2005) 583–590.

[15] S. Inzucchi, et al., Insulin-sensitizing antihyperglycemic drugs and mortality after acute myocardial infarction: insights from the National Heart Care Project, Diabetes Care 28 (2005) 1680–1689.

International Congress Series 1303 (2007) 160 – 171

www.ics-elsevier.com

Lifestyle and outcome among patients with type 2 diabetes

Gang Hu [a,b,*], Jaakko Tuomilehto [a,b,c]

[a] *Department of Health Promotion and Chronic Diseases Prevention, National Public Health Institute, Helsinki, Finland*
[b] *Department of Public Health, University of Helsinki, Helsinki, Finland*
[c] *South Ostrobothnia Central Hospital, Seinäjoki, Finland*

Abstract. Type 2 diabetes is one of the fastest growing public health problems in both developed and developing countries. Cardiovascular disease is the most prevalent complication of type 2 diabetes. Data from prospective studies have shown that regular physical activity is an efficient tool in the prevention of cardiovascular disease events in type 2 diabetic patients. The favorable association of physical activity with longevity was observed regardless of the levels of body mass index, blood pressure, total cholesterol, and smoking. Several dietary factors modify the risk of type 2 diabetes, and also the risk of cardiovascular disease in patients with diabetes. For instance coffee drinking reduces the risk of type 2 diabetes in the population, and furthermore in type 2 diabetic patients it is associated with a decreased risk of cardiovascular risk. Results from clinical trials have indicated that lifestyle changes, including dietary modification and increase in physical activity, can prevent type 2 diabetes. Public health messages, health care professionals, and the health care system should strongly promote physical activity and healthy nutritional habits during daily life and prevent overweight and obesity. Prevention of cardiovascular disease in patients with type 2 diabetes should start from the prevention of diabetes itself. © 2007 Published by Elsevier B.V.

Keywords: Diabetes; Cardiovascular disease; Lifestyle factor; Physical activity; Diet

1. Introduction

Diabetes is one of the fastest growing public health problems in both developing and developed countries [1]. It has been estimated that the number of individuals with diabetes

* Corresponding author. Department of Health Promotion and Chronic Diseases Prevention, National Public Health Institute, Helsinki, Finland. Tel.: +358 919127366; fax: +358 919127313.
E-mail address: hu.gang@ktl.fi (G. Hu).

0531-5131/ © 2007 Published by Elsevier B.V.
doi:10.1016/j.ics.2007.03.022

among adults 20 or more years of age will double from the current 171 million in 2000 to 366 million in 2030 [1]. Much of the burden of diabetes is attributable to microvascular and macrovascular complications, such as retinopathy, nephropathy, coronary heart disease (CHD), and stroke. Cardiovascular disease (CVD) accounts for more than 70% of total mortality among patients with type 2 diabetes [2]. Epidemiological studies have indicated that patients with type 2 diabetes have a 2–4 times higher risk of CVD mortality than those without diabetes [3,4]. In addition, CVD mortality among diabetic subjects without prior myocardial infarction (MI) is similar to non-diabetic subjects with prior MI at baseline [5]. One recent study reports that in men, MI at baseline or during follow-up means a greater risk of coronary mortality than diabetes does; in women, prior MI at baseline is associated with a lower risk of coronary mortality than prior diabetes, but incident MI during follow-up is associated with a greater risk than incident diabetes [6]. Moreover, mortality after the first MI is higher in patients with diabetes than their non-diabetic counterparts [7].

Lifestyle factors, such as diet, physical activity and obesity, have a major influence on the development and progression of the conditions that precede the onset of type 2 diabetes and subsequent complications. The prevalence of unhealthy lifestyle factors, such as inactivity and obesity, and their negative health consequences are rapidly increasing in the world [8,9]. Physical inactivity, unhealthy diet and obesity have been estimated to account for about 14% of all deaths in the United States [10,11]. According to conservative estimates, physical inactivity accounts for about 4% and obesity for about 7% of direct health care costs in the United States, figures that are comparable to those related to smoking [12]. Modification of lifestyle factors is an important strategy for reducing the incidence of type 2 diabetes and subsequent complications. In this review, we summarize the current information about the role of increased exercise and nutritional factors in the prevention and management of CVD among patients with type 2 diabetes.

2. Physical activity and the risk of CVD mortality among patients with type 2 diabetes

There is good evidence that regular physical activity reduces the risk of CVD in the general population [8,13]. Recently, several studies have assessed the association between physical activity or physical fitness and the risk of CVD mortality among patients with type 2 diabetes [14–20]. The results from the Aerobic Center Longitudinal Study [14], the Nurses' Health Study [15], the Whitehall Study [16], the National Health Interview Survey [17], and the Health Professionals' Follow-up Study [18] have indicated that regular leisure-time physical activity is associated with reduced CVD and total mortality among patients with diabetes or impaired glucose tolerance. Walking has a similar inverse association with the risk of cardiovascular and total mortality to that of vigorous leisure-time physical activity [15–18]. In the Aerobic Center Longitudinal Study, physical fitness had a strong and independent inverse association with total mortality in men with diabetes, and this association was seen in all body mass index and body fatness group [14,19].

The analyses from the FINMONICA study also evaluated whether other types of physical activities, such as occupational and daily commuting physical activity on foot or by bicycle, are related to reduced cardiovascular mortality among diabetic patients [20]. We reviewed data on 3316 patients aged 25 to 74 with history of type 2 diabetes who participated in surveys of randomly selected samples from the Finnish population

Table 1
Hazard ratios of cardiovascular mortality according to occupational, commuting and leisure-time physical activity among Finnish patients with type 2 diabetes [20]

	Deaths, *n*	Person-years	Hazard ratios (95% CIs)[a]	
			Model 1	Model 2
Occupation physical activity				
Light	517	25,549	1.00	1.00
Moderate	161	13,216	0.84 (0.70–1.01)	0.91 (0.75–1.10)
Active	225	22,305	0.59 (0.50–0.69)	0.60 (0.50–0.71)
P for trend			<0.001	<0.001
Walking or cycling to and from work				
0 min	609	33,530	1.00	1.00
1–29 min	165	15,581	0.81 (0.67–0.96)	0.89 (0.75–1.07)
≥30 min	129	11,959	0.74 (0.61–0.90)	0.86 (0.70–1.06)
P for trend			0.002	0.27
Leisure-time physical activity				
Low	480	27,974	1.00	1.00
Moderate	381	28,072	0.85 (0.74–0.98)	0.83 (0.72–0.95)
High	42	5024	0.70 (0.51–0.96)	0.67 (0.49–0.93)
P for trend			0.016	0.005

[a] Model 1: adjusted for age, sex, study year, body mass index, systolic blood pressure, cholesterol and smoking; model 2, adjusted also for other two physical activity.

conducted between 1972 and 1997. The data included questionnaires on the level of physical activity on the job; on the way to and from work; and during their leisure time. During an average follow-up of 18.4 years, 1410 of the subjects died, 903 (64%) from cardiovascular disease. After adjusting for age, gender, body mass index, systolic blood pressure, total cholesterol, smoking and the other two categories of physical activity, we found that moderately active work was associated with a 9% reduction in cardiovascular mortality and active work was associated with a 40% reduction (Table 1). High level of leisure-time physical activity was associated with a 33% drop and moderate activity was linked to a 17% drop in cardiovascular mortality compared with the most sedentary group. Daily walking or cycling to and from work decreased cardiovascular mortality, but this relation was no longer significant after additional adjustment for occupational and leisure-time physical activity.

We further merged and regrouped these three types of physical activity into three categories: low was defined as subjects who reported light levels of occupational, commuting (<1 min) and leisure-time physical activity; moderate was defined as subjects who reported only one of the all three types of moderate to high physical activity; high was defined as subjects who reported two or three types of moderate to high physical activity. We found that those who were moderately active reduced their risk of dying from cardiovascular disease by 39%, while those who were highly active reduced the risk by 48% (Table 2) [21]. The protective benefits of physical activity were consistent regardless of body mass index, blood pressure or cholesterol levels or whether or not the person smoked (Table 3) [21]. Thus, American Diabetes Association, the National Cholesterol Education Program Export Panel and International Diabetes Federation (European Region) have recommend physical activity

Table 2
Hazard ratios of cardiovascular mortality according to different levels of physical activity, body mass index, blood pressure, total cholesterol, and smoking among Finnish participants with type 2 diabetes [21]

	Deaths, *n*	Person-years	Hazard ratios (95% CIs)	
			Model 1[a]	Model 2[b]
Physical activity				
Low	264	10,940	1.00	1.00
Moderate	304	21,437	0.60 (0.51–0.71)	0.61 (0.52–0.73)
High	338	36,781	0.49 (0.41–0.58)	0.52 (0.44–0.62)
Body mass index (BMI)[c]				
Tertile 1	249	24,358	1.00	1.00
Tertile 2	313	23,575	1.04 (0.88–1.23)	1.00 (0.84–1.18)
Tertile 3	344	21,225	1.38 (1.17–1.62)	1.22 (1.03–1.44)
Diastolic blood pressure[c]				
Tertile 1	221	20,751	1.00	1.00
Tertile 2	271	23,232	0.94 (0.78–1.12)	0.89 (0.74–1.07)
Tertile 3	414	25,175	1.36 (1.15–1.61)	1.29 (1.08–1.54)
Systolic blood pressure[c]				
Tertile 1	198	23,896	1.00	1.00
Tertile 2	266	22,714	1.07 (0.89–1.29)	1.06 (0.88–1.28)
Tertile 3	442	22,548	1.60 (1.35–1.90)	1.55 (1.30–1.84)
Total cholesterol[c]				
Tertile 1	217	20,888	1.00	1.00
Tertile 2	297	23,923	1.04 (0.87–1.24)	1.05 (0.88–1.26)
Tertile 3	392	24,347	1.19 (1.00–1.41)	1.20 (1.01–1.43)
Smoking status				
Never	499	39,147	1.00	1.00
Former	167	10,576	1.01 (0.81–1.25)	1.01 (0.81–1.26)
Current	240	19,434	1.35 (1.12–1.63)	1.34 (1.11–1.63)

[a] Model 1: adjusted for age, sex, and study year.

[b] Model 2 included the following variables: for physical activity: age, sex, study year, education, BMI, systolic blood pressure, total cholesterol, and smoking; for BMI: age, sex, study year, education, physical activity, systolic blood pressure, total cholesterol, and smoking; for diastolic and systolic blood pressure: age, sex, study year, education, physical activity, BMI, total cholesterol, and smoking; for cholesterol: age, sex, study year, education, physical activity, BMI, systolic blood pressure, and smoking; for smoking: age, sex, study year, education, physical activity, BMI, systolic blood pressure, and total cholesterol.

[c] Cutpoints for tertile of BMI were 27.1 and 30.4 kg/m^2 in men, 28.0 and 32.6 kg/m^2 in women; cutpoints for tertile of diastolic blood pressure were 88 and 98 mm Hg in men, 87 and 98 mm Hg in women; cutpoints for tertile of systolic blood pressure were 141 and 158 mm Hg in men, 144 and 165 mm Hg in women; cutpoints for tertile of total cholesterol were 5.8 and 6.9 mmol/l in men, 6.0 and 7.0 mmol/l in women.

for the primary and second prevention of cardiovascular complications among patients with type 2 diabetes [22–24].

3. Coffee consumption and risk of CVD mortality among patients with type 2 diabetes

There are dietary factors that may increase the risk of type 2 diabetes while some others may decrease the risk [25]. Diabetes increases the risk of cardiovascular disease. This risk is modified by several dietary and lifestyle factors, some may increase while others may reduce the risk. Higher habitual coffee drinking has been associated with a lower risk of

Table 3
Hazard ratios of cardiovascular mortality according to joint levels of physical activity, body mass index, blood pressure, total cholesterol, and smoking among Finnish participants with type 2 diabetes [21]

	Hazard ratios (95% CIs)	
	Active[a]	Inactive[a]
Body mass index (BMI)[b]		
Tertile 1	1.00	1.74 (1.28–2.37)
Tertile 2	1.01 (0.83–1.23)	1.68 (1.29–2.18)
Tertile 3	1.21 (1.00–1.46)	2.23 (1.76–2.81)
Diastolic blood pressure[c]		
Tertile 1	1.00	2.05 (1.53–2.74)
Tertile 2	0.96 (0.78–1.20)	1.55 (1.17–2.04)
Tertile 3	1.35 (1.10–1.66)	2.45 (1.89–3.16)
Systolic blood pressure[c]		
Tertile 1	1.00	2.36 (1.74–3.22)
Tertile 2	1.18 (0.95–1.48)	1.87 (1.38–2.52)
Tertile 3	1.72 (1.40–2.12)	2.85 (2.21–3.67)
Total cholesterol[d]		
Tertile 1	1.00	1.66 (1.24–2.23)
Tertile 2	0.99 (0.80–1.22)	1.94 (1.48–2.54)
Tertile 3	1.19 (0.97–1.46)	2.01 (1.56–2.58)
Smoking status[e]		
Never	1.00	1.89 (1.56–2.29)
Former	1.05 (0.83–1.34)	1.75 (1.22–2.51)
Current	1.43 (1.16–1.77)	2.22 (1.65–2.99)

[a] Inactive was defined as low physical activity; active was defined as moderate or high physical activity.
[b] Adjusted for age, sex, study year, education, systolic blood pressure, total cholesterol, and smoking.
[c] Adjusted for age, sex, study year, education, BMI, total cholesterol, and smoking.
[d] Adjusted for age, sex, study year, education, BMI, systolic blood pressure, and smoking.
[e] Adjusted for age, sex, study year, education, BMI, systolic blood pressure, and total cholesterol.

developing type 2 diabetes [26–28]. The relation between coffee consumption and risk of CVD has been examined in many studies in cohorts based on general populations, but the issue remains controversial [29–32]. Is it not known whether coffee consumption influences the risk of CVD in diabetic patients, and if it does, to which direction? The analyses from our group assessed the association between coffee consumption and the risk of total, CVD, coronary heart disease (CHD) and stroke mortality among Finnish patients with type 2 diabetes [33].

The study comprised 3837 randomly ascertained Finnish patients with type 2 diabetes aged 25 to 74 years. Coffee consumption was determined at baseline survey. During the average follow-up of 20.8 years, 1471 deaths were recorded, of which 909 were coded as CVD, 598 as CHD and 210 as stroke. The respective multivariate-adjusted hazard ratios in participants who drank 0–2, 3–4, 5–6, and ≥7 cups of coffee daily were 1.00, 0.77, 0.68 and 0.70 for total mortality ($P<0.001$ for trend), 1.00, 0.79, 0.70 and 0.71 for CVD mortality ($P=0.006$ for trend), 1.00, 0.78, 0.70 and 0.63 for CHD mortality ($P=0.01$ for trend), and 1.00, 0.77, 0.64 and 0.90 for stroke mortality ($P=0.12$ for trend) (Table 4). This study showed an inverse association between coffee consumption and the risk of total, CVD, and CHD mortality among a population-based sample of patients with type 2 diabetes. These associations were

Table 4
Hazard ratios for of total, cardiovascular, coronary heart disease, and stroke mortality by volume of coffee consumption among Finnish subjects with type 2 diabetes [33]

	Daily coffee consumption (cups/day)				*P* for trend
	0–2	3–4	5–6	≥7	
Total mortality	1.00	0.77 (0.65–0.91)	0.68 (0.58–0.80)	0.70 (0.59–0.85)	<0.001
Cardiovascular mortality	1.00	0.79 (0.64–0.97)	0.70 (0.57–0.86)	0.71 (0.56–0.90)	0.006
Coronary heart disease mortality	1.00	0.78 (0.60–1.01)	0.70 (0.54–0.90)	0.63 (0.47–0.84)	0.01
Stroke mortality	1.00	0.77 (0.50–1.19)	0.64 (0.41–0.99)	0.90 (0.56–1.45)	0.12

Adjusted for age, sex, study year, body mass index, systolic blood pressure, total cholesterol, education, alcohol and tea consumption, and smoking status.

independent of age, body mass index, systolic blood pressure, total cholesterol, physical activity, alcohol drinking and smoking. Research into potential health effects of coffee in this population is of particular interest since Finns have the highest per capita coffee consumption (11.4 kg/year) in the world.

Most probable mechanisms involved are the antioxidant activity of coffee's components and their effect on the different stages of glucose metabolism, leading to improved control of hyperglycaemia. Also reduced inflammation may be involved as indicated in the recent study [34]. However, investigations in other populations are required in order to confirm the findings of an inverse association between coffee consumption and CVD mortality among diabetic patients.

4. Other lifestyle factors (obesity and smoking) and risk of CVD mortality among patients with type 2 diabetes

Overweight and obesity are currently recognized as important risk factors for atherosclerotic CVD and premature mortality [9,35]. Prospective epidemiological studies have consistently shown that overweight and obesity are associated with an increase risk of CHD and CHD among general population. Overweight and obesity predict CHD in both men and women [36–43]. Abdominal obesity has been found to be a stronger risk factor for CHD than overall obesity in men and women and may provide additional information beyond overall obesity in the prediction of CHD [39,40,44–48].

However, the association between obesity and CVD mortality among diabetic patients is controversial and only few prospective studies have evaluated this association. The results from the United Kingdom Prospective Diabetes Study indicated that high levels of body mass index and waist to hip ratio were not major risk factors for CHD among diabetic patients [49]. The direct association between body mass index and mortality among men with diabetes was found in the Aerobics Center Longitudinal Study, however, this association became non-significant when fitness was accounted for [19]. We recently found that diabetic patients with obesity, defined as the highest tertile of body mass index, had a higher risk of CVD mortality than those in the lowest tertile of body mass index after controlling for many other potential risk factors (Table 2) [21]. This direct association was consistent in diabetic patients with different levels of physical activity (Table 3).

Epidemiological prospective studies have shown that smoking is one of most important risk factors for CHD among general populations [50]. Several studies have indicated that smoking was an independent predictor of CVD mortality also in diabetic patients [19,49,51,52]. We found that current smoking was associated with increased CVD mortality among patients with type 2 diabetes (Table 2) and this association was observed among patients with different levels of physical activity (Table 3) [21].

Patients with type 2 diabetes should avoid excessive alcohol consumption. Moderate alcohol consumption with food does not appear to adversely affect blood glucose or insulin levels, and alcohol can be considered as part of a meal plan for patients with diabetes [53].

5. Preventing progression to diabetes: early intervention in high-risk individuals

Lifestyle factors such as poor diet with excessive energy intake and a sedentary lifestyle, which in turn lead to obesity, have a major impact on the risk of developing type 2 diabetes [54,55]. In recent years, several clinical trials have assessed whether regular physical activity, with or without dietary intervention, can reduce progression to type 2 diabetes among adults with impaired glucose tolerance [56–60] and among men with high cardiovascular risk [61].

The Malmö study from Sweden targeted increased physical exercise and weight loss as major intervention strategies to prevent and delay type 2 diabetes [56]. Subjects with impaired glucose tolerance had less than half the risk of developing type 2 diabetes during the 5-year follow-up, compared with those who did not take part in the exercise program. In the Chinese study from Da Qing, 577 individuals with impaired glucose tolerance were allocated to clinics randomized into one of the four groups: exercise only, diet only, diet plus exercise, and a control group [57]. The cumulative incidence of type 2 diabetes during 6 years was significantly lower in the exercise group (41%), diet group (44%), and diet plus exercise group (46%), compared with the control group (68%), and remained significant even after adjusting for differences in baseline body mass index and fasting glucose.

In the Finnish Diabetes Prevention Study (DPS), 522 middle-aged (mean age 55 years) men (33%) and women (67%), who were overweight (mean body mass index 31 kg/m^2) and had impaired glucose tolerance, were randomized either to an intensive lifestyle intervention group or a control group [58,62]. The subjects in the intervention group had frequent consultation visits with a nutritionist (seven times during the first year). They received individual advice about how to achieve the intervention goals, including 1) reduction in body weight of 5% or more, 2) total fat intake less than 30% of energy consumed, 3) saturated fat intake less than 10% of energy consumed, 4) fiber intake of at least 15 g per 1000 kcal, and 5) moderate exercise for at least 30 min per day. After the intensive intervention period, there was a maintenance phase that included a counseling session every 3 months. At each of these counseling sessions, exercise habits were discussed, all kinds of physical activity were strongly recommended, and increased physical activity was considered an essential part of successful weight loss program [63]. Endurance exercise, including walking, jogging, swimming, aerobic ball games, and skiing, was recommended to increase aerobic capacity and cardiorespiratory fitness. Participants were also offered an opportunity to attend supervised, progressive, individually tailored circuit-type resistance training sessions. The moderate intensity and medium to high volume programs were designed to improve the functional capacity and strength of the large muscle groups of the upper and lower body. The cumulative incidence of type 2 diabetes after 4 years was 11% in the intervention group and 23% in the control group. During the entire trial, the risk of diabetes was reduced by 58% in the intervention group. The reduction in the incidence of diabetes was directly associated with changes in lifestyle, since few of the people who reached four or five of the five lifestyle targets developed diabetes. However, with a multifactorial intervention study design it is not possible to point out a single factor that could be called the primary reason for the reduced risk of developing diabetes since all changes in healthy lifestyle are important, and in different people different lifestyle changes matter more than others. This can be due to the lifestyle patterns, but also genetic factors can play a role in the response to the lifestyle changes [64].

Recently, the Finnish DPS researchers further assessed the extent to which the originally-achieved lifestyle changes and risk reduction remain after discontinuation of active counselling in the extended follow-up [65]. After a median of 4 years of active intervention, participants who were still free of type 2 diabetes were further followed up for a median of 3 years. Beneficial lifestyle changes achieved by participants in the intervention group were maintained after the discontinuation of the intervention, and the corresponding incidence rates during the post-intervention follow-up were 4.6 and 7.2 per 100 person-years, indicating still a 36% further reduction in the relative risk of diabetes during the period when no intervention was no longer provided.

A similar randomized clinical trial of lifestyle change and the risk of developing type 2 diabetes among persons at high risk, the Diabetes Prevention Program (DPP), was conducted in the United States. In the DPP, 3234 non-diabetic persons with elevated fasting and post-load plasma glucose concentrations were randomized to a placebo group, a group assigned metformin, or a group assigned a lifestyle-modification program with the goals of at least a 7% weight loss and at least 150 min of physical activity per week [59,66]. The mean age of the participants was 51 years, the mean body mass index was 34.0 kg/m^2, 68% of the participants were women, and 45% of them were members of non-Caucasian ethnic groups. The exercise intervention emphasized brisk walking, but other activities with equivalent intensity, including aerobic dance, bicycle riding, skating, and swimming, were also recommended. The participants were advised to distribute their physical activity throughout the week, with at least 10 min per session. Voluntary, supervised physical activity sessions were offered at least twice per week throughout the study, including group walks, aerobic classes, and one-to-one personal training. After an average follow-up of 2.8 years, the incidence of diabetes was 11.0, 7.8 and 4.8 cases per 100 person-years in the placebo, metformin and lifestyle groups, respectively. The lifestyle intervention reduced the incidence by 58% and metformin by 31%, compared with placebo, and the lifestyle intervention was significantly more effective than metformin in the prevention of type 2 diabetes.

In the Indian Diabetes Prevention Program, 531 individuals with impaired glucose tolerance were randomized into four groups: a group assigned metformin, a group assigned to a lifestyle-modification, a group assigned to both lifestyle-modification and metformin, and a control group [60]. The cumulative incidence of type 2 diabetes during the median follow-up period of 30 months was significantly lower in the lifestyle-modification group (39%), the metformin group (41%), and the lifestyle-modification plus metformin group (40%), compared with the control group (55%).

In the 1970s, the Multiple Risk Factor Intervention Trial (MRFIT) in the United States enrolled 12,866 middle-aged men 35–57 years of age at a high risk for coronary heart disease and delivered either special intervention or usual care over 6–7 years [61]. This trial, initiated in 1973, was originally designed to examine coronary heart disease as the outcome of interest. The special intervention group was counseled to change diet by reducing saturated fat, cholesterol, and calorie intake, to stop smoking, and to increase physical activity. Recently, the data from the MRFIT were used to investigate the role of the lifestyle intervention program in preventing type 2 diabetes. In 11 827 men without diabetes and impaired fasting glycemia at baseline, a total of 666 men (11.5%) in the special intervention group and 616 men (10.8%) in the usual care group met the criteria for diabetes during 6 years of follow-up. Among nonsmokers, the intervention program resulted in a statistically significant 18% reduction in the incidence of diabetes compared with the usual care group. In smokers, however, diabetes risk in the intervention group increased significantly by 26%. While smoking is clearly a significant risk factor for type 2 diabetes [67], it is not know how to reduce the risk of diabetes in smokers [68].

6. Conclusion

Diabetes is one of the fastest growing public health problems in the world, and it is a major economic, social and personal burden. A variety of organizations, including the Centers for Disease Control and Prevention, the American College of Sports Medicine [8], the National Institutes of Health of the United States [69] and the World Health Organization [70] have suggested that every adult should have at least 30 min moderate-intensity physical activity (such as brisk walking, cycling, swimming, home repair, and yard work) on most, preferably all, days of the week. Our review based on the scientific evidence is consistent with this recommendation, and confirms that regular physical activity, avoiding excessive weight gain, and a healthy diet are effective and safe ways to prevent CVD events in type 2 diabetic patients. Regular physical activity and a healthy weight are important components of health lifestyle for all of us. Public health messages, health care professionals, and health care system should aggressively promote physical activity during occupation, commuting, leisure time and daily life and prevent overweight and obesity. This is not only a task for health personnel, but they should take a lead in the process towards the primary prevention of type 2 diabetes and subsequent complications.

Acknowledgement

This study was supported by the Finnish Foundation for Cardiovascular Research.

References

[1] S. Wild, et al., Global prevalence of diabetes: estimates for the year 2000 and projections for 2030, Diabetes Care 27 (5) (2004) 1047–1053.

[2] M. Laakso, Hyperglycemia and cardiovascular disease in type 2 diabetes, Diabetes 48 (5) (1999) 937–942.

[3] G. Assmann, H. Schulte, The Prospective Cardiovascular Munster (PROCAM) study: prevalence of hyperlipidemia in persons with hypertension and/or diabetes mellitus and the relationship to coronary heart disease, Am. Heart J. 116 (6 Pt 2) (1988) 1713–1724.

[4] J. Stamler, et al., Diabetes, other risk factors, and 12-yr cardiovascular mortality for men screened in the Multiple Risk Factor Intervention Trial, Diabetes Care 16 (2) (1993) 434–444.

[5] S.M. Haffner, et al., Mortality from coronary heart disease in subjects with type 2 diabetes and in nondiabetic subjects with and without prior myocardial infarction, N. Engl. J. Med. 339 (4) (1998) 229–234.
[6] G. Hu, et al., The gender-specific impact of diabetes and myocardial infarction at baseline and during follow-up on mortality from all causes and coronary heart disease, J. Am. Coll. Cardiol. 45 (9) (2005) 1413–1418.
[7] H. Miettinen, et al., Impact of diabetes on mortality after the first myocardial infarction. The FINMONICA Myocardial Infarction Register Study Group, Diabetes Care 21 (1) (1998) 69–75.
[8] R.R. Pate, et al., Physical activity and public health. A recommendation from the Centers for Disease Control and Prevention and the American College of Sports Medicine, JAMA 273 (5) (1995) 402–407.
[9] World Health Organisation, Obesity: prevention and managing the global epidemic, WHO Technical Report Series, vol. 894, World Health Organization, Geneva, 2000.
[10] J.M. McGinnis, W.H. Foege, Actual causes of death in the United States, JAMA 270 (18) (1993) 2207–2212.
[11] D.B. Allison, et al., Annual deaths attributable to obesity in the United States, JAMA 282 (16) (1999) 1530–1538.
[12] G. Colditz, A. Mariani, The costs of obesity and sedentarism in the United States, in: C Bouchard (Ed.), Physical Activity and Obesity, Human Kinetics, Champaign, IL, 2000, pp. 55–65.
[13] S.G. Wannamethee, A.G. Shaper, Physical activity in the prevention of cardiovascular disease: an epidemiological perspective, Sports Med. 31 (2) (2000) 101–114.
[14] M. Wei, et al., Low cardiorespiratory fitness and physical inactivity as predictors of mortality in men with type 2 diabetes, Ann. Intern. Med. 132 (8) (2000) 605–611.
[15] F.B. Hu, et al., Physical activity and risk for cardiovascular events in diabetic women, Ann. Intern. Med. 134 (2) (2001) 96–105.
[16] G.D. Batty, et al., Physical activity and cause-specific mortality in men with Type 2 diabetes/impaired glucose tolerance: evidence from the Whitehall study, Diabet. Med. 19 (7) (2002) 580–588.
[17] E.W. Gregg, et al., Relationship of walking to mortality among US adults with diabetes, Arch. Intern. Med. 163 (12) (2003) 1440–1447.
[18] M. Tanasescu, et al., Physical activity in relation to cardiovascular disease and total mortality among men with type 2 diabetes, Circulation 107 (19) (2003) 2435–2439.
[19] T.S. Church, et al., Exercise capacity and body composition as predictors of mortality among men with diabetes, Diabetes Care 27 (1) (2004) 83–88.
[20] G. Hu, et al., Occupational, commuting, and leisure-time physical activity in relation to total and cardiovascular mortality among Finnish subjects with type 2 diabetes, Circulation 110 (6) (2004) 666–673.
[21] G. Hu, et al., Physical activity, cardiovascular risk factors, and mortality among Finnish adults with diabetes, Diabetes Care 28 (4) (2005) 799–805.
[22] National Institute of Health, Executive Summary of The Third Report of The National Cholesterol Education Program (NCEP) Expert Panel on Detection, Evaluation, And Treatment of High Blood Cholesterol In Adults (Adult Treatment Panel III), JAMA 285 (19) (2001) 2486–2497.
[23] American Diabetes Association, Physical activity/exercise and diabetes mellitus, Diabetes Care 26 (1 Supple) (2003) S73–S77.
[24] Working Party of the international Diabetes Federation (European Region), Hypertension in people with Type 2 diabetes: knowledge-based diabetes-specific guidelines, Diabet. Med. 20 (12) (2003) 972–987.
[25] N.P. Steyn, et al., Diet, nutrition and the prevention of type 2 diabetes, Public Health Nutr. 7 (1A) (2004) 147–165.
[26] J. Tuomilehto, et al., Coffee consumption and risk of type 2 diabetes mellitus among middle-aged Finnish men and women, JAMA 291 (10) (2004) 1213–1219.
[27] R.M. van Dam, F.B. Hu, Coffee consumption and risk of type 2 diabetes: a systematic review, JAMA 294 (1) (2005) 97–104.
[28] G. Hu, et al., Joint association of coffee consumption and other factors to the risk of type 2 diabetes: a prospective study in Finland, Int. J. Obes. (Lond.) 30 (12) (2006) 1742–1749.
[29] S. Greenland, A meta-analysis of coffee, myocardial infarction, and coronary death, Epidemiology 4 (4) (1993) 366–374.
[30] P. Kleemola, et al., Coffee consumption and the risk of coronary heart disease and death, Arch. Intern. Med. 160 (22) (2000) 3393–3400.
[31] P. Happonen, S. Voutilainen, J.T. Salonen, Coffee drinking is dose-dependently related to the risk of acute coronary events in middle-aged men, J. Nutr. 134 (9) (2004) 2381–2386.
[32] E. Lopez-Garcia, et al., Coffee consumption and coronary heart disease in men and women: a prospective cohort study, Circulation 113 (17) (2006) 2045–2053.

[33] S. Bidel, et al., Coffee consumption and risk of total and cardiovascular mortality among patients with type 2 diabetes, Diabetologia 49 (11) (2006) 2618–2626.
[34] L.F. Andersen, et al., Consumption of coffee is associated with reduced risk of death attributed to inflammatory and cardiovascular diseases in the Iowa Women's Health Study, Am. J. Clin. Nutr. 83 (5) (2006) 1039–1046.
[35] Overweight, obesity, and health risk. National Task Force on the Prevention and Treatment of Obesity, Arch. Intern. Med. 160 (7) (2000) 898–904.
[36] J.E. Manson, et al., A prospective study of obesity and risk of coronary heart disease in women, N. Engl. J. Med. 322 (13) (1990) 882–889.
[37] E.B. Rimm, et al., Body size and fat distribution as predictors of coronary heart disease among middle-aged and older US men, Am. J. Epidemiol. 141 (12) (1995) 1117–1127.
[38] W.C. Willett, et al., Weight, weight change, and coronary heart disease in women. Risk within the 'normal' weight range, JAMA 273 (6) (1995) 461–465.
[39] K.M. Rexrode, et al., Abdominal adiposity and coronary heart disease in women, JAMA 280 (21) (1998) 1843–1848.
[40] A.R. Folsom, et al., Associations of general and abdominal obesity with multiple health outcomes in older women: the Iowa Women's Health Study, Arch. Intern. Med. 160 (14) (2000) 2117–2128.
[41] A.E. Field, et al., Impact of overweight on the risk of developing common chronic diseases during a 10-year period, Arch. Intern. Med. 161 (13) (2001) 1581–1586.
[42] K.M. Rexrode, J.E. Buring, J.E. Manson, Abdominal and total adiposity and risk of coronary heart disease in men, Int. J. Obes. Relat. Metab. Disord. 25 (7) (2001) 1047–1056.
[43] T.Y. Li, et al., Obesity as compared with physical activity in predicting risk of coronary heart disease in women, Circulation 113 (4) (2006) 499–506.
[44] B. Larsson, et al., Abdominal adipose tissue distribution, obesity, and risk of cardiovascular disease and death: 13 year follow up of participants in the study of men born in 1913, Br. Med. J. 288 (6428) (1984) 1401–1404.
[45] P. Casassus, et al., Upper-body fat distribution: a hyperinsulinemia-independent predictor of coronary heart disease mortality. The Paris Prospective Study, Arterioscler. Thromb. 12 (12) (1992) 1387–1392.
[46] A.R. Folsom, et al., Body fat distribution and 5-year risk of death in older women, JAMA 269 (4) (1993) 483–487.
[47] W.Y. Fujimoto, et al., Visceral adiposity and incident coronary heart disease in Japanese-American men. The 10-year follow-up results of the Seattle Japanese-American Community Diabetes Study, Diabetes Care 22 (11) (1999) 1808–1812.
[48] H.M. Lakka, et al., Abdominal obesity is associated with increased risk of acute coronary events in men, Eur. Heart J. 23 (9) (2002) 706–713.
[49] R.C. Turner, et al., Risk factors for coronary artery disease in non-insulin dependent diabetes mellitus: United Kingdom Prospective Diabetes Study (UKPDS: 23), BMJ 316 (7134) (1998) 823–828.
[50] P. Jousilahti, et al., Sex, age, cardiovascular risk factors, and coronary heart disease: a prospective follow-up study of 14 786 middle-aged men and women in Finland, Circulation 99 (9) (1999) 1165–1172.
[51] A.R. Folsom, et al., Prediction of coronary heart disease in middle-aged adults with diabetes, Diabetes Care 26 (10) (2003) 2777–2784.
[52] W.K. Al-Delaimy, et al., Smoking and risk of coronary heart disease among women with type 2 diabetes mellitus, Arch. Intern. Med. 162 (3) (2002) 273–279.
[53] M.J. Franz, et al., Evidence-based nutrition principles and recommendations for the treatment and prevention of diabetes and related complications, Diabetes Care 26 (Suppl 1) (2003) S51–S61.
[54] T. Costacou, E.J. Mayer-Davis, Nutrition and prevention of type 2 diabetes, Annu. Rev. Nutr. 23 (2003) 147–170.
[55] G. Hu, et al., Occupational, commuting, and leisure-time physical activity in relation to risk for type 2 diabetes in middle-aged Finnish men and women, Diabetologia 46 (3) (2003) 322–329.
[56] K.F. Eriksson, F. Lindgarde, Prevention of type 2 (non-insulin-dependent) diabetes mellitus by diet and physical exercise. The 6-year Malmo feasibility study, Diabetologia 34 (12) (1991) 891–898.
[57] X. Pan, et al., Effects of diet and exercise in preventing NIDDM in people with impaired glucose tolerance. The Da Qing IGT and Diabetes Study, Diabetes Care 20 (4) (1997) 537–544.
[58] J. Tuomilehto, et al., Prevention of type 2 diabetes mellitus by changes in lifestyle among subjects with impaired glucose tolerance, N. Engl. J. Med. 344 (18) (2001) 1343–1350.
[59] W.C. Knowler, et al., Reduction in the incidence of type 2 diabetes with lifestyle intervention or metformin, N. Engl. J. Med. 346 (6) (2002) 393–403.

[60] A. Ramachandran, et al., The Indian Diabetes Prevention Programme shows that lifestyle modification and metformin prevent type 2 diabetes in Asian Indian subjects with impaired glucose tolerance (IDPP-1), Diabetologia 49 (2) (2006) 289–297.
[61] G. Davey Smith, et al., Incidence of type 2 diabetes in the randomized multiple risk factor intervention trial, Ann. Intern. Med. 142 (5) (2005) 313–322.
[62] J. Eriksson, et al., Prevention of Type II diabetes in subjects with impaired glucose tolerance: the Diabetes Prevention Study (DPS) in Finland. Study design and 1-year interim report on the feasibility of the lifestyle intervention programme, Diabetologia 42 (7) (1992) 793–801.
[63] J. Lindstrom, et al., The Finnish Diabetes Prevention Study (DPS): Lifestyle intervention and 3-year results on diet and physical activity, Diabetes Care 26 (12) (2003) 3230–3236.
[64] V.I. Lindi, et al., Association of the Pro12Ala polymorphism in the PPAR-gamma2 gene with 3-year incidence of type 2 diabetes and body weight change in the Finnish Diabetes Prevention Study, Diabetes 51 (8) (2002) 2581–2586.
[65] J. Lindstrom, et al., Sustained reduction in the incidence of type 2 diabetes by lifestyle intervention: follow-up of the Finnish Diabetes Prevention Study, Lancet 368 (9548) (2006) 1673–1679.
[66] The Diabetes Prevention Program Research Group, The Diabetes Prevention Program (DPP): description of lifestyle intervention, Diabetes Care 25 (12) (2002) 2165–2171.
[67] K. Patja, et al., Effects of smoking, obesity and physical activity on the risk of type 2 diabetes in middle-aged Finnish men and women, J. Intern. Med. 258 (4) (2005) 356–362.
[68] J. Tuomilehto, Primary prevention of type 2 diabetes: lifestyle intervention works and saves money, but what should be done with smokers? Ann. Intern. Med. 142 (5) (2005) 381–383.
[69] NIH Consensus Development Panel on Physical Activity and Cardiovascular Health, Physical activity and cardiovascular health. NIH Consensus Development Panel on Physical Activity and Cardiovascular Health, JAMA 276 (3) (1996) 241–246.
[70] World Health Organisation, Global strategy on diet, physical activity, and health, Report No.: WHA27.17, Agenda Item 12.6, 2004 Geneva.

Author index

Keyword index

www.ingramcontent.com/pod-product-compliance
Ingram Content Group UK Ltd.
Pitfield, Milton Keynes, MK11 3LW, UK
UKHW051027041026
15470UKWH00015B/1641

9 780444 528896